My Heart Attack Saved My Life ... But for What?

Follow one woman's path to discover how change can bring you freedom

Susan Smith

Copyright © 2023 Susan Smith
Print Edition

ISBN eBook: 979-8-9885581-0-1
ISBN Print: 979-8-9885581-1-8

Heart Smart Press
Written by Susan Smith
Book development and editing by Milli Thornton
Author photo courtesy Tricia Turpenoff
Cover Design by Alexander von Ness • www.nessgraphica.com
Photos: Pixabay.com
Interior design by BB eBooks

All rights reserved. This book or parts thereof may not be reproduced in any form, stored in any retrieval system, or transmitted in any form by any means—electronic, mechanical, recording or otherwise—without prior written permission of the publisher, except as provided by United States of America copyright law. For permissions, write to the publisher at the email address below.

The insights presented in this book should not be considered as a replacement for a balanced lifestyle, proper self-care, your doctor's advice, or professional counsel wherever warranted.

Author's website:
susansmithheart.com

To contact the author:
susan@susansmithheart.com

*For my husband, Tomas,
my sons, Tim and Nathan,
and my grandsons, Patrick and Devin.
I love you so much. You make my heart sing.*

TABLE OF CONTENTS

Acknowledgments	vii
PART ONE: WHAT RED FLAG?	**1**
You Can't Do Anything If You're Dead	5
Feeling the Breeze on My Face	10
Sleeping While Praying	13
PART TWO: ENFORCED CHANGE	**19**
Outperforming Myself	23
Looking for the Real Me	26
The Call to Change	35
The Challenge to Change	39
The Nature of Change	41
Simple Tools for Change	46
PART THREE: HEY, I'M LEARNING	**51**
Losing Heart	55
Filling the Half-Empty Glass	63
The Power of Choice	73
Multitasking My Life Away	82
Resistance Is Futile	88
Control vs. Flow	92
PART FOUR: PIVOTING	**101**
People Pleaser	105
The Power of Getting Help	110

PART FIVE: WHAT'S A HEART REALLY FOR?   117
Miles of Smiles   121
Joie de Vivre   127
My Inner Kid   134
Rewarding My Heart   140

PART SIX: THE TRUE SELF   147
Heart in Nature   151
If My Heart Ruled the World   155
The Heart's Wisdom   159

About the Author   165
Interviews & Heart Health Resources   167

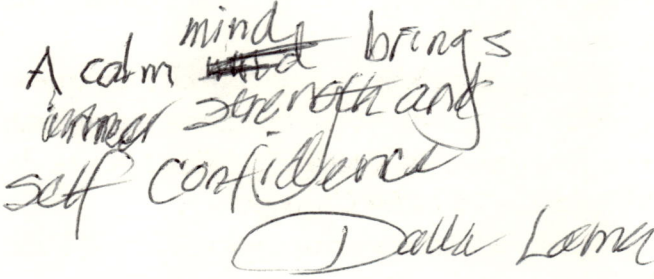

ACKNOWLEDGMENTS

I could not have finished this book without the help of my book coach, Milli Thornton, and her gentle encouragement. Her superpower is practicing deep acknowledgment. She's adept at recognizing not only what I've done, but who I am—my qualities and characteristics—keeping me confident and actively writing. I've never written so much! The words just pour out of me. With her strong intuition and knack for crafting writing assignments, I love Milli's ability to keep me creating.

I'd also like to thank Milli in her capacity as guest writer. Her contribution was vital for these important chapters: "The Challenge to Change," "The Nature of Change," and "Simple Tools for Change."

I'd like to warmly thank my writer friends, Pam Hale Trachta and Susan Luzader. Over the course of 30 years, Pam and Susan have helped me revise and edit essays, articles, and book chapters. We attended and taught writing classes together, learning and writing all the way. Their devotion to the written word motivates me to write.

I want to thank another special writer friend, Lori DiGuardi. From the day I met her, I knew I had a writing buddy. Lori's dedication to her books and her writing uplifts and inspires me. She generously offers sage advice, and she introduced me to Milli, my book coach.

Profound thanks to my husband, Tomas, who read every draft of every chapter. For health fairs and my speaking engagements, Tomas is the one who makes sure I have the right people watching me like a hawk. He takes them aside and says, "Make sure she eats, hydrates, and doesn't stand too long." He knows me so well. And he cares about this book as much as I do.

Finally, I want to express my appreciation for my son, Tim Bentley. In the years since my heart attack, Tim has become a life coach for me. On so many occasions, his calm words and easy approach to life keep me from jumping back into my busy-bee lifestyle. He gives me great ideas, sensible advice, and valuable insight. Tim's the one who coined my life mantra, #justbe.

If this is the *only* disclaimer you ever read

. . . it may someday save your life.

If you suspect you're having a medical emergency, call 911 NOW. Don't let the fear of a "false alarm" stop you from getting the help you need.

In reading this book, you assume full responsibility for your own health and how you choose to use this information. This book is not a substitute for professional medical advice.

> Robert Fulghum wrote a great essay about a guy who was dying and decided not to tell his family because he didn't want to worry them. Fulghum compared this to the one kid who plays hide-and-seek a little too well. He says he wants to shout, "Get found, kid!"
> —Rachel Whalley

PART ONE

WHAT RED FLAG?

Catch on fire if you must. Sometimes everything needs to burn to the ground so that we may grow.
—A. J. Lawless

You Can't Do Anything If You're Dead

Women experience heart attacks differently than men. Men have the "Hollywood" attacks we see in movies: pain in the left arm, clutching the chest, collapsing.

I had none of those signs.

But I did have signs.

I was scheduled to be the spotlight speaker for one of my networking groups. Because I'd done this compelling talk before, I knew it would convince people to sign up for my writing class.

At six-thirty that morning, I began preparing for my talk. My fingers and toes were icy cold. I was tired and hadn't been sleeping well, but I'd been chalking it up to any number of things: a poor dinner choice the night before, a case of nerves, or maybe sleep apnea.

I began packing up my handouts and props. I still needed to make copies and find business cards. I also needed to gather crayons and drawing paper for the coloring exercise. As I wrote my speech notes onto blue index cards, I was breathless. My collarbone ached as if it were being pinched.

I planned to arrive at the lunch meeting at eleven o'clock to set up my props. While loading the supplies into my SUV, I noticed I was winded even from that level of effort.

The meeting was being held at a local restaurant. At the restaurant, tables were set up in a hollow square formation to accommodate forty or more people. I took an end seat so I could get up easily to do my presentation. I heard the buzz of conversation around me and noticed my mouth was dry. I asked the waiter for some water.

The microphone came out. The leader explained it wasn't working well. He instructed us to hold it tightly and put it directly in front of our mouths when we spoke. I watched as others struggled to get through their 30-second elevator speeches without the mic crackling or cutting out.

It was my turn. I stood at the front—all eyes were on me—and laid out my note cards in front of me. Then I grasped the microphone for dear life.

Despite the static coming from the mic, I talked easily for ten minutes, though I realized I was getting short of breath. I dismissed it as speaking too quickly or forgetting to breathe between sentences.

My heart started pounding. This was (I thought) probably because I was holding my breath—until it pounded faster, and I mean *really* pounded. It took everything I had to appear calm and composed. After all, I was giving a speech!

I started feeling lightheaded, to the point of dizziness. While the group got busy on the crayon exercise, I clutched the back of a chair to steady myself. I relaxed my tight grip on the microphone, breathed deeply, and tried to regain my composure. I walked around the square of tables, looking at the drawings people were making. This seemed to calm my heart.

At the end of my time, I took a few questions and sat down just before the room started to spin. Immediately, sweat formed at my hairline and trickled down my forehead, like a menopausal hot flash. I dabbed at my forehead with a napkin, desperate to be "fine."

A friend noticed that all the color had drained from my face. She brought me more water. The waiter brought me Sprite. They wanted to call 911, but I resisted.

"No! I'm fine. Just feeling a bit woozy. . . ."

I figured I'd been standing for too long, hadn't eaten my lunch—a hundred excuses!

I sensed I might pass out, and I wanted to lie down, but there was nowhere I could do that.

I kept saying, "I'm fine. Honest, I'm fine." Finally, after drinking lots of water and using more napkins to mop up the cold sweat pouring from my scalp, I felt somewhat recovered.

Knowing I couldn't drive in this condition, I called my husband to come and take me home. There, I lay on the couch, very still, and googled my symptoms. *Anxiety attack.* That explained everything! Somehow, this made me feel better, even though I couldn't imagine what I might have been anxious about. But anxiety *had* to be it.

I rested, ate dinner, and went to bed, confident I'd be fine the next day.

* * *

Friday, February 9, 2018.

I awoke with a head full of plans and a long to-do list. Among other things, I needed to go to the grocery store to buy food and snacks for my writing class on Saturday.

First, though, I wanted to get cleaned up. In the shower, raising my arms to wash my hair felt like such an effort. I was quickly out of breath. With a towel wrapped around my head, I put on my fuzzy robe and lay down on the bed until my breathing returned to normal.

Blow-drying my hair caused the same effect. So, back to bed I went, lying down for the second time that morning—and it wasn't even eight o'clock. My thoughts raced.

This is unacceptable. I have too much to do to be lying down every five minutes!

Determined to push through and prepare for my Saturday writing class, I charged off to the grocery store. I knew exactly where to find all my favorite foods for the class. Veggie tray, crackers, cheese, fruit... but in the cookie aisle, it hit me. I reached for a pack of gourmet cookies, and they fell to the floor. As I bent down to retrieve them, I knew I'd faint if I leaned all the way down.

I left the cookies on the floor and retreated to the register to check out.

My legs felt so heavy, I could barely move. Thinking a jolt of sugar and caffeine would pick me up, I grabbed a cold soda and gulped it down.

As if moving through syrup, I slowly loaded my bags of groceries into the back of the SUV. I was short of breath again, and the pain in my collarbone was now constant.

After I got home, I finally gave in and called my primary care doctor.

"Sorry, he's out of town," said the nurse who answered the phone.

"Is someone covering for him? Who can I see?"

Her answer was short.

"Call your cardiologist. Or go to the nearest emergency room."

"I can't go to the ER," I wailed. "I have too much to do!"

Her reply haunted me for months.

"You can't do anything if you're dead."

Feeling the Breeze on My Face

Thankfully, I did have a cardiologist to call. It had been ten years since my last visit, but the receptionist found my file. She told me the doctor could work me in at one o'clock that day. I called my husband Tomas and we drove there together.

Soon I was hooked up to an EKG. The tech shook his head as he watched the needle move. The associate doctor came in, looked at the machine, and frowned. Dr. Marshall, the head doctor, entered the room. As they all stared at the machine, I knew something was up.

Dr. Marshall looked at me. "Susan, you're having a heart attack."

What?

It can't be.

I thought he would just give me blood pressure pills and send me on my way.

Terrified, I looked over at my husband. Tomas looked terrified, too.

"You need to go to the ER—NOW."

Things happened fast.

The tech gave me a baby aspirin, and the associate doctor gave me nitroglycerin under my tongue. I heard Dr. Marshall on the phone swiftly making arrangements for me.

Oh, God, I prayed silently.

DAY ONE

Tomas drove me to Tucson Medical Center's ER entrance, which was only four blocks from the doctor's office. I was whisked inside and placed on a gurney. I winced as the attendant peeled off my brand-new black leggings and my underwear. I was allowed to take off my top and bra myself. The hospital gown went on so quickly that nobody saw me naked.

The cardiac team swarmed around me.

Doctors, nurses, and techs each announced their names and what they would be doing to me. Calmly, they took my blood, put in a needle for an IV, asked about my health history and medications—and my nail polish.

Yes, my nail polish. They wanted to remove it so they could clip an oxygen monitor onto my finger. They said the polish would interfere, but I knew it wouldn't come off because it was made of shellac. I tried to explain this but to no avail. Instead, they quickly attached the monitor to my ear.

I felt a breeze on my face from the speed of the moving gurney. As they rolled me to somewhere called the cardiac catheterization laboratory, one of the nurses explained what that meant. "It's an exam room where doctors will use tiny flexible tubes called catheters to look at the arteries of your heart." Having received anesthesia, I didn't care.

In the cath lab, I was surrounded by nurses, equipment, and blinking monitors. The doctor threaded a tiny wire with a balloon on the end through a catheter tube in my groin. From there, he inserted a stent into my circumflex artery. It was 95 percent blocked and resistant to opening but, with the stent in place, my blood flow improved to 60 percent.

Less than twenty minutes had passed since arriving in the ER.

Sleeping While Praying

When I woke up from the anesthesia, I found myself in a private room with nurses, techs, and orderlies coming in and out. My husband was there, and so was my son Tim.

I was starving, but I couldn't eat until another round of tests had been run. That night was a blur of fitful sleep, bad dreams, a dinner tray at ten o'clock, and a constant struggle to get comfortable.

DAY TWO

The early morning ushered in more nurses, who got busy drawing blood, bringing pills, and taking my vitals. My breathing was still labored, and my collarbone pain had moved to my chest.

Three doctors visited and determined I wasn't better, so they ordered a few tests. They gave me something for the pain, and to get the fluid off my lungs, then sent me off for a chest x-ray. After that, I was wheeled out on yet another gurney for an echocardiogram, a test that uses ultrasound to evaluate one's heart muscle and valves.

Hours later, Dr. Waggoner, the hospital's cardiologist, told me he was taking me back to the cath lab to fix another artery with a stent. I trusted him. I knew something had to be done because I felt so bad—

constant chest pains, shortness of breath, fitful sleep, and non-stop sweating. I had also noticed the nurses' frowns of concern whenever they took my blood pressure and checked my monitors.

After receiving a second stent, I improved dramatically.

The second stent opened up the right coronary artery, improving the blood flow along with oxygen to my body. My test results improved. Everyone noticed!

This fix marked the beginning of a slow recovery as my heart began to grow stronger.

DAY THREE

By the third day after my heart attack, my brain was on overload, trying to take in every face, test result, and procedure explanation. I had three cardiologists, four nurses, a dietician, a pharmacist, a physiologist, and a hospitalist who managed my case. One nurse was a counselor who had a soothing voice and wore a fuzzy cardigan.

Dr. Peña, my hospitalist, visited me every day. He'd squat down to look me in the eye, hold my hand, and ask if I knew what had been happening to me. His soft voice calmed me. He made sure I knew I'd had a heart attack and then stent surgery procedures. Whatever the circumstance, he took care to explain the details to me.

Sarah, the nurse with the fuzzy cardigan, told me, "Because you almost died, you'll find yourself feeling depressed. Just expect this to happen at some point."

A kid in blue scrubs—a cardiac rehab intern—said he'd walk me down the hall to see how far I could go. This excited me! I wanted to prove I was strong enough to be released. He offered his arm, and we started our walk. I made it a few steps out the door of my room before I was so winded I had to stop. My ankles felt wobbly, and my legs felt weak.

Then came Debbie, a manufacturer's rep dressed in a slim skirt and peplum jacket. I wanted her to meet my bachelor son, she was that cute. Her job was to explain how to use a contraption I was supposed to wear 24/7 for six weeks. She opened a color brochure and showed me a defibrillator vest.

The vest was like a fabric sports bra with metal paddles in the back. Debbie explained that if a dangerous arrhythmia were to be detected by the sensors, the device would sound an alarm. If I failed to respond to the alarm within one minute, the paddles would deliver a shock, restoring normal rhythm to my heart.

Because it was Sunday, I wouldn't get the actual vest until Monday.

The dietician lady wearing red scrubs was sweet as she launched into long explanations of what I should be eating for the rest of my life. Her visual of the desired salt intake mesmerized me. "Just make a little mound about the size of a dime in the palm of your hand," she said. "That's how much salt you can have in a day. Not just from the salt shaker but from *everything* you eat." Then she showed me how to read labels on food products, especially the sodium content.

Cradling the stack of brochures she'd given me, I felt woozy and my eyelids were drooping. "This is a lot to take in," I murmured.

Before I drifted off, I heard my doctor speaking with Tomas about the "ejection fraction," or EF numbers. EF is a measure of how well the left ventricle is pumping blood. With a normal heart putting out 50 to 70 percent, mine was very low at 15 percent. This explained the need for a defibrillator vest.

I ordered heart-healthy chicken soup for dinner, but it tasted like dishwater. Yuck, no salt. I craved salt badly, so I ate the saltine crackers. I dozed off again and later heard the clicking of heels in my room. Opening my eyes, I saw my best friend bearing a vase of flowers.

"Happy birthday," she said.

"Diana," I blurted. "I told you not to come!"

"I had to see you with my own eyes to make sure you were okay."

That's when I started to cry. I didn't want anyone to see me looking so debilitated—oxygen tube, catheter bag, tubes and needles in both arms, bruises on every visible surface.

I wanted to tell her I had almost died and how scared I was, but my breathing was so labored I couldn't get the words out. We simply hugged.

DAY FOUR

Finally, Monday morning came, and so did a flurry of activity.

A young man in gray scrubs went through my discharge paperwork. One by one, he explained what the points meant so I could knowledgeably sign the papers. Most important was understanding the long list of drugs, their names, dosages, and what they would do for me.

It felt like a barrage: *Do this, do that, make an appointment for this doctor, that blood test.*

A chipper nurse dressed in brown corduroy came next, carrying my new defibrillator vest. With great enthusiasm, she showed me the first step for how to put it together, by inserting the electrodes, also known as paddles, into their proper slots. Then the skinny black cords were to be threaded through the waistband so that the sensors—all eight of them—would touch my body through the thin fabric.

"Put it on and get me out of here!" I wanted to shout. But no, I'd have to prove to her that I could put it together. Like a puzzle, she disconnected the parts, then made me put them back in place while she watched.

Despite my resistance, I knew that any slacking off on my part would be unwise. Wearing this vest was serious, life-saving stuff.

The kid in scrubs came to walk with me again. This time I made it farther than before. I wanted to jump for joy, but I couldn't let go of his arm.

DAY FIVE: FIRST NIGHT AT HOME

Tomas and I decided I should sleep in the guest room and keep the walker nearby. I would need it when I got up to go to the bathroom. I wasn't strong enough to make it there on my own.

That night, I had a nightmare, awoke with a start, and began to hyperventilate. My breath wouldn't come. I was terrified. I made my way to the family room, got into the recliner, and covered myself with an afghan. I could breathe better sitting up.

While in that chair, I had a long talk with God.

"Please help me breathe better right now!" I wheezed.

My eyelids fluttered open. I kept them at slits and saw fuzzy shapes in the room. My breathing felt slow and steady.

"God, thank you for hearing my prayer!"

I touched my forehead with two fingers as if to stave off a headache. I felt softer and looser.

"And thank you for sparing my life. What can I do to repay you for saving me?"

I fell asleep mid-prayer.

PART TWO

ENFORCED CHANGE

I became an overachiever to get approval
from the world.
—Madonna

Outperforming Myself

> I have to admit, I was dismayed when I found out "Type A" refers to the risk of heart disease. I thought it was just a nickname my mom gave me!
> —Reese Witherspoon

One time I decided to list all my groups, meetings, classes, and clubs, along with the meeting days, in the back of my day planner. In my organized manner, I divided them by type: women's groups, networking clubs, charity organizations, lunch groups with friends, online courses, and mastermind groups. There were easily 20 items on the list.

My calendar was packed with weekly and monthly meetings and a few quarterly gatherings. Some days I'd have a lunch meeting and an evening event. No problem!

Then there was my digital world.

By the time Zoom became the norm during the COVID-19 shutdown, I'd been attending Zoom meetings for several years. Some women hated them, but I was plenty comfortable with meetings conducted on Zoom. It allowed me to attend meetings of my favorite professional women's group anywhere in the country. There's a chapter in nearly every state.

I also became connected to a leader who offered women sure-fire ways to become entrepreneurs working from anywhere in the world. It didn't matter what your business was—or even whether you had a business yet. Her name was Monica, and she taught us her tips for getting customers and doing business online.

My product was an online course centered around writing one's life story. I had developed a method to get a writer thinking, remembering, and creating pieces from her lifetime. This would become a memoir.

I learned from Monica about the "best" software to use to set up an online course. I learned about marketing in an "automatic" way. I was posting every day on Instagram, Facebook, and LinkedIn. Everything had a schedule.

Before I knew it, people were asking me to do anything but help them write their life story.

First there was Deanne, a petite brunette who owned and ran a preschool. "I've already written the story of my unique childhood," she said. "Will you read it and tell me what you think?" I asked Deanne to send me a chapter so I could assess her project. Oh my, it was so disjointed. Too many storylines and characters.

Next was Lorna. An elegant 60-something dressed in Chanel, she approached me at a meeting. "I have a beautiful love story in my head. It's the story of how I met my husband. I think it would make a great screenplay. Can you help me put my idea together and find a producer?"

Another off-target request came from a serious, dark-haired young woman named Connie. "I don't want to follow a system. Can you just coach me through writing my book and finding a publisher?"

I said yes to all comers and let them know my hourly rate was fifty dollars. Even though I knew I was in over my head, I found myself creating services for editing, screenwriting, and book coaching—including publishing.

* * *

About a week after the heart attack, my son Tim helped me announce to my circles that I was out of commission. We canceled two writing workshops and refunded the fees. I closed two private Facebook groups where I'd been offering a weekly writing prompt. I stopped posting on social media. We let everyone know I didn't have the energy for phone calls.

No more networking; no more crazy posting schedules; no more drained energy. I took two naps per day and went to cardiac rehab for a workout.

I gave up every group except for my women's networking group. This filled my cup, offering a talented national speaker, a wonderful lunch, and some much-needed camaraderie. For these outings, I asked a good friend to sit with me, to make sure I ate and stayed hydrated, and to keep me from lingering too long. We joked that she was my "handler."

Apart from this tiny oasis of freedom, I dutifully stayed home and rested. Like a prisoner with a ball and chain, I faithfully wore the life vest.

But this wasn't the real me.

Looking for the Real Me

> Words mean nothing when your actions contradict.
> —Anonymous

I loved meeting with women who were heart attack survivors and needed to talk.

Janet was only 42. "When I had a heart attack," she said during our first call, "I didn't know what happened. They sent me home without any instructions." She began to sniffle. "I went back to work a week later."

"What?!" I exclaimed, gripping my cell phone more tightly.

"My husband thought that, since I had stents, I was as good as new." More sniffling. "One day I was so tired, I collapsed on the bed and slept for three hours. He came home and asked me what I was doing."

"Needing an afternoon nap is very common after a heart attack," I offered in a reassuring tone. "Your heart is healing and needs all of your body's energy for the job."

"That's the point. I have zero energy. I don't know what to do."

"Did they send you to cardiac rehab?"

"To what?" she asked.

Oh my, I thought privately.

"Are you working tomorrow? Your work is not far from me. Why don't I come by and we can talk."

"Oh, yes, please. I have so many questions."

The next day I walked into a lovely lobby with high ceilings and lush sofas. The tall windows allowed sunshine to nourish rows of thriving green plants. I dialed her cell phone number.

"I'm here. I'll wait in the lobby."

A pretty young woman with curly brown hair approached me. "Susan?"

I popped up from the sofa. "Yes, it's me."

"I'm so glad you came." We hugged. "Let's sit over here," she added, as she pulled me to another cushy sofa in a private corner.

"Thank you for coming!" Janet burst into tears. "I don't know anyone with experience I can talk to."

"I can help you with that. We have a women's support group with plenty of heart attack survivors." I handed her a folder. "Here's some literature from WomenHeart about women and heart disease."

I watched her shaky hands as she answered her cell phone.

"I'm just in the lobby. Yes, meeting with a client."

She ended the call. "I don't think I can keep this up. I'm thinking about quitting and taking disability."

"What's stopping you?" I asked.

"They don't have anyone to replace me."

I looked into her eyes, recognizing the symptoms. "You're a giver, aren't you?"

"I guess so," she said, gulping tears again, "but I can't just leave them shorthanded."

"I don't mean to get bossy," I said, "but it's time you start taking care of you. I'll help. First, let's get you into cardiac rehab. Can you take three days off?"

"Yes, why?"

"So we can plan your self-care recovery." I handed her the paperwork to get into my favorite cardiac rehab gym. "Have your cardiologist sign this and fax it in. I know you'll be accepted. Set up sessions at least twice a week. Your heart will get stronger, and so will you."

"Okay," she said softly.

"After you do that, call and tell me the days you're taking off. In the meantime, I want you to write down everything, every day."

Janet blinked. "I don't know if I can write that much."

"You'll feel better after clearing your head. Think of it as journaling, a way of putting all your feelings and questions on paper. Then make a list of things you consider self-care. Email me when you have 10 things."

"Why?"

"We'll put together a list of activities and routines you can do during your three days off. Things just for you."

Janet has a beautiful smile. I saw it engulf her entire face when she said, "I feel better already. Can I call you when I feel low?"

"Of course. Anytime."

• • •

My mother-in-law was turning 100, and we were going to the birthday party. In the car, I complained to Tomas.

"The party lasts all day. I don't know why we had to leave so early!"

"I promised we'd come at ten o'clock to help set up," Tomas said, glancing sideways at me with *that* look.

On the long dirt driveway to Joey's pink stucco house, clouds of dust roiled behind the CRV.

"We don't have to speed, you know," I grumbled. "We have the whole day."

In the silence Tomas responded with, I prayed for the wind to die down.

"Why is it always so windy in Sierra Vista? The wind makes it impossible to be outside."

He gave me another sideways look.

"Okay, I'll stop whining. It's just that we've been driving for nearly two hours."

"Let's put our best faces on," he said, finally slowing down. "A lot of relatives traveled a long way to celebrate with her." Parking at the side of the garage, he added sternly, "Don't get out until I get there."

Tomas pushed his hat down hard on his head to keep the wind from whipping it off. Opening the passenger door, he handed me my cane. I wrinkled my nose.

"You really should have this. It might be crowded."

Treading gingerly on the narrow sidewalk, I stopped and took a deep breath. "I want to go in behind you."

The front porch was long. A low overhang was shading a cluster of relatives.

"Pam's here," he said, cluing me in on names I may have forgotten. "And there's Susan and Barbara, the cousins from Alabama."

"Oh, you made it!" exclaimed brother Shawn. "We thought you weren't coming."

I gave Shawn a hug. "We figured out a way to make it work. How's my favorite brother-in-law?"

Putting my smile on, I told Tomas, "I'm going inside. Maybe I can find Martha." I opened the screen door and called down the narrow hallway. "Where's the birthday girl?"

No answer.

Tripping on the step up into the house, I righted myself, whispering, "Good catch, Susan."

Tripping is something I've had to learn to take more seriously. The two life-saving artery stents I received in 2018 were only the beginning of a long journey back to health. This journey was marked by more health scares, including several more heart procedures and a mini-stroke.

Seemingly out of nowhere, I'd had a series of falls, including a serious one, and started physical therapy. PT is routine for falls among the elderly. It took almost six months before the mini-stroke was indicated by a dark spot on my brain during an MRI. As part of balance therapy, the physical therapist taught me how to catch myself when falling.

Tripping again on one of the many rugs, I grabbed the back of a heavy wooden dining room chair.

"Darn it!" I sat heavily, plopping on the only free chair at the table. "Where's the birthday girl?"

A cousin chimed in. "She's holding court in the back guest room."

I maneuvered my way down the bedroom hallway, watching my step for trip hazards. Laughter erupted from the back room.

"You girls are having too much fun!" I said to the room. "Hi, Martha."

Martha looked up and squinted. "Come closer, so I can see you."

I went to Martha's chair and squatted down so we were eye to eye. "It's me, Susan," I said, taking her hand.

"I'm so glad you came!" Martha said, with a big grin. "I thought you weren't able to come. Are you feeling better?"

Squeezing her hand and noticing how cold it was, I said, "I wouldn't miss your big birthday bash for anything."

Sunshine filtered through the mini-blinds, burnishing her silvery hair and reflecting from her glasses.

"Why don't I take you out to the sunroom?" I said brightly. "People are waiting to see you. Let me get your walker."

Martha grasped the handles with all her might. "Ha!" I said. "We make quite the pair—you in your walker, me with my cane."

We both fell silent as we concentrated on the narrow hallway.

Martha planted herself on the sofa. "Let's get you cozy," I said, wrapping a soft blanket around her shoulders.

"Oh, that feels nice." Martha smiled up at me.

Later, after a whirlwind of socializing, my husband touched my shoulder. "Do you want to go to lunch? We're thinking of the Mexican restaurant in town."

In the car, Tomas sounded relieved. "I can't visit one more minute without eating."

"That was a lot of people," I commented. "I don't know why I'm so tired already."

"You should be ready for your two o'clock nap after lunch. Right?"

"I'm not *that* tired! Just hungry. Lunch will perk me up."

Tomas sighed.

"Susan, you promised. We agreed you would take your regular nap, so we could stay the entire day."

I just looked out the window.

Gordo's restaurant was packed. I raised my voice slightly. "This crowd is a good sign. The food must be great! Smells delicious."

* * *

As we were driving back to the party, I received a text from Joey.

"Hope you're on your way. The American Legion motorcycle flag ceremony is set for two o'clock."

Smiling, I turned to Tomas. "We'd better hurry, or we're going to miss the fun."

"Susan. . . ." he started.

"Honey, I'll be fine."

The porch was still crowded. "Excuse us," I said, as I pushed my way through the chattering throng. Pulling the front screen door open, I called, "Joey, we're back!"

She came out of the kitchen. Pushing her hair off her face with the back of her hand, she said, "I'm so glad you're here. I need help serving the cake."

"Sure! Where are the plates?"

"Just use these paper plates," she ordered.

Winding my way through the crush, I carried four plates at once. I addressed those standing around: "Want some cake? Big piece or small?"

As I worked the room for a third time, Martha grabbed my arm. "Where's mine?"

I handed her the last one in my stash. "Here you go. A special piece just for you."

She beamed at me.

With my cake duties discharged, I was glad to find an empty chair. I sat heavily and let a sigh escape.

"You're tired, aren't you?" Pam questioned.

"Not me!" I gave her my most professional smile.

But, secretly, I was sweating from my scalp. The pinching in my collarbone got my attention.

"Excuse me," I said oddly, to the table of strangers. "I'm going to the bathroom."

In the bathroom, I got down on the floor, put my feet up on the lid of the toilet, and took five deep breaths. "Come on," I said, ordering the dizziness to go away.

Eventually feeling better, I returned to the room.

"Anybody need anything?"

A heavy-set man said, "I could use some coffee and another piece of cake."

"Sure thing," I said breezily.

I got busy serving the guests.

Later, Shawn said, "We're leaving now. The kids have an early flight in the morning."

Almost like a bell had been rung, departure time spread through the house. As people began filing through the front door, Joey said, "Who's taking Martha home?"

I raised my arm and opened my mouth. Tomas clapped me on the shoulder.

"No!" His whisper was harsh in my ear. "Someone else can do it. Come on, let's go. It's nearly six."

After more goodbyes, hugs, and promises to keep in touch, I felt Tomas pulling me out the front door. I couldn't resist one last farewell. "Bye, everybody!" I said to the thinning crowd on the porch.

As we made our way to the car, I was leaning on Tomas. My legs were so heavy that I could barely lift my feet. I was moving at the speed of a tortoise.

"I'm really tired. I can't feel my legs."

Tomas spoke quietly. "You know what happens when you miss your nap." I was surprised he didn't sound angry. "Let's get you home."

In the car, I opted not to mention my side trip to the bathroom, but silently I was hard on myself.

You should stop thinking you can just push through and not suffer the consequences.

At home, Tomas said, "Let me get you to bed." As if wading through quicksand, I let him guide me. "I won't wake you up in the morning. You just sleep in."

The next day, I didn't get out of bed at all. My inner voices were chattering.

Why did you push yourself to do more? the one I call Critical Cathy gloated.

"I couldn't help it. They needed my help."

The Call to Change

> Change is hard. You fight to hold on. You fight to let go. But in the end, we all know. Change is needed for you to grow.
> —Nishan Panwar

I saw her name on the caller ID. Jacqueline Donner Powell.

"Hello, Jackie. How are you?"

"I hope I'm not interrupting you." Her smooth voice lulled me. "I'm working on next year's calendar and want to make sure we have you speaking in February for Heart Month."

Jacqueline is a tall, elegant woman with flawless skin. An aura of success surrounds her. Many call her Miss Jackie. It's a matter of respect.

"Sure! I'd be glad to, Miss Jackie," I bubbled. "But I'd better put something new together."

"The message never gets old," she said. "And your story is the kind our audience needs to hear."

"I'll put it on my calendar!"

After the call was over, I felt anxious and elated at the same time.

"I've booked my first speaking gig in two years," I told my husband with a radiant smile. "It's not till February next year."

Tomas raised an eyebrow. "Didn't you say you were going to avoid those? You know how much they drain you."

"This'll be a piece of cake. It's my favorite group, filled with friends. I'll be relaxed."

I paused, lifting my chin in thought. "Except . . . I'll have to make a new PowerPoint and update the statistics in my speech. And I should address how COVID-19 affects heart patients."

"Don't overdo," he warned.

One day, as I was sorting Christmas decorations, I thought about my upcoming heart talk. It had been three months since I'd promised Jackie I would speak in February.

"Oh, darn," I said to the air. "I'll have to update that entire presentation. I'd better call Tim."

One foot jiggled anxiously as I dialed his number. "Hi, Tim, it's Mom," I said into his voicemail. "I was hoping you could help me update my PowerPoint for my heart talk. Call me!"

Tim didn't just call, he came in person. As we discussed the details of my speech, my real feelings surfaced.

"I'm not feeling fully recovered after my stroke," I said, staring at my shoes. "I don't know if I can stand for an hour giving this talk."

"Mom, why did you accept? Maybe you can get someone else to do it."

The more I thought about creating a new presentation, gathering new statistics, and practicing the speech, the more anxious I became.

Now it was January, just one month before the scheduled speaking date. I dialed Miss Jackie's number. When I heard her voice, I almost lost my nerve.

"I have some bad news," I said. "I realize I cannot speak at your February meeting. I have some health issues to resolve."

* * *

Psychotherapist Cynthia Goddard greeted me with a welcoming smile. "Hello, Susan."

I took a seat on a vintage Woodard patio chair. Brick pavers covered the ground of her peaceful patio. Bougainvillea and wisteria vines were entwined along the stucco walls, filling the space with a delicious flowery scent.

Cynthia sat across from me, dressed in linen pants and a silk blouse. Her hair was highlighted and cut in a classic shoulder-length bob. She had a French manicure, which I couldn't help but notice as she talked with her hands.

As I shared my feelings, her hand gestures underscored the most important points.

"I'm pissed off. My body isn't doing what I want it to do. I can't believe this is happening to me. It's been *four years* since the heart attack, and I can't get back to normal!"

I couldn't stop my rant. "I get tired in the afternoon and have to take a nap like a toddler. And, guess what? A brain scan found a mini-stroke. I didn't even know I'd had it!"

I took a breath, trying to compose myself.

"Why am I so mad? I don't get it. It doesn't even suit my personality."

Cynthia's hands stopped in midair.

"I believe you're suffering from grief. Being angry is one of the stages in the grief process. Denial is another."

She explained that I was still grieving my old lifestyle, my former, well-functioning body, and the abundant energy from past years. "Grief takes time to overcome. There's no quick fix."

My jaw went slack. *Oh, crap, I think she's right.*

I put my forehead in my hands as I processed her diagnosis.

Understanding the Nature of Change

The Challenge to Change

> After nourishment, shelter, and companionship, stories are the thing we need most in the world.
> —Philip Pullman

If you're anything like me, you've read more than your fair share of self-help books.

Maybe you've also tried a range of other things: meditating, repeating positive affirmations, listening to guided audios, attending self-development seminars, and so on. Maybe you've joined support groups or tried sessions with energy healers.

If yes, why is it still so hard to change in some stubborn area of your life?

I've come to see that what's needed before we push ourselves to change is *an understanding of the nature of change*. This is rarely mentioned, and yet it can be crucial to your success. The chapter that follows this one will go into more depth about the nature of change.

What's also needed is to approach yourself at the right level. Where is change being resisted the hardest? Deep down in the unconscious mind—that wild place where you seem to have little or no conscious influence. However, when approached in the right way, the unconscious mind can process harmlessly.

And that approach is something simple. Something you already enjoy.

I'm talking about stories.

We're all hungry for good stories. We love stories in movies and novels, from our own lives and the lives of others. We love hearing them, watching them, reading them, and telling them. No matter what else has changed down through history, stories have been with us since ancient times. There's a good reason for that. Stories reach us deep inside. It's a primitive thing.

However, as writer and history-making judge Albie Sachs noted, "Primitive does not mean stupid."

Why would a "primitive" approach work? I'm not a psychoanalyst but, as a storyteller, here's my take on it: While your conscious mind is busy feeling engaged with what you're reading, stories allow your unconscious mind to acknowledge tough emotions.

I hope you'll enjoy the variety of stories I've prepared for you. These stories came from my own life experiences.

Some will remind you how a simple thing can be life-changing.

Some will show how your heart can make you happy, if you remember to let it.

Other stories portray how I handled certain situations the hard way, eventually arriving at a friendlier destination. I call those my Before & After stories.

The Nature of Change

> The secret of change is to focus all your energy
> not on fighting the old, but on building the new.
> —Dan Millman

When you desire to change something about yourself or your life, an understanding of the nature of change can be vital to your success. Here are some aspects of the nature of change that you may find helpful.

To be truly effective and lasting, change has to come from within.

You may have heard this many times before, but what does it mean, exactly?

Changing from within means getting in tune with your real self. When you're out of whack with your own deepest needs and desires, this inevitably creates repercussions—such as making choices that turn out to be wrong for you.

Getting in tune with yourself doesn't have to be complicated. In fact, your inner self may be trying to show you something at any time. Getting more in tune can be as simple as putting awareness on feelings that surface from inside of you.

Is there something you're about to take on that's giving you a nagging feeling? Get in tune with your real self by allowing yourself to notice that feeling.

Intention matters.
You can read my stories just for fun. Or you can learn more about yourself as you read. Either way is great. It all depends on what you want.

If you do want to let your deeper self speak, mentally say something to this effect: *I'd like to discover more about myself as I read*. This is a way of giving your inner self permission.

Change can be simple.
You've heard about how people manage to make things harder than they need to be. You've seen others do it (and it's painful to watch). And you know what it feels like when you catch yourself doing it.

Even sticky notes stuck all over the house saying "Keep it simple!" can fail to bring change.

This time, there are no "failures." This time, I encourage you to do something different: acknowledge that change can be simple. That's all. Just say it to yourself: "Change can be simple."

This will set up an intention inside of you. As you read this book (or perhaps as you go about your day), suddenly you'll have an "Aha" moment. You'll spot something you've been doing that could be a lot simpler. It will pop into your awareness, and you'll feel relief at recognizing it.

If that Aha moment doesn't happen today, trust that it will happen at the right moment—probably when you've forgotten all about it.

Don't force it by trying to find something you can simplify *right now*. That would defeat the elegance of letting your inner self easefully help you—the epitome of simple.

Remember, all you have to do to prime your inner self is to say, "Change can be simple."

Change is progressive.

Change isn't always straightforward. As you contact deeper layers of it, you may keep revisiting an issue over time. And that's when you may get discouraged.

Didn't I already deal with this? Why is this back? What am I doing wrong?

Cycles of change keep happening until the change is fully assimilated. Each time you go through a cycle, you make progress. I know, sometimes it can feel like regressing! However, as long as you're consciously aware of the pattern when it comes up again, you'll be making progress.

Your own self-awareness is more powerful than you think.

Change is challenging, so be patient with yourself. Encourage yourself.

In your adult self, you already know this. But, when it comes to change, you're not dealing only with the conscious, adult part of yourself. You're dealing with what some call the inner child. That's the part of you that can seem unreasonable or irrational when it "regresses" because it holds so many unresolved feelings.

Whenever you're getting frustrated that your life is not changing at the speed you want it to, remember a moment when someone encouraged you, and what a difference that made. Being patient and encouraging with yourself can be life-changing.

One caveat. If you are a trauma survivor, please seek out the proper support. Please don't rely merely on a book. Don't try to go it alone.

If you go off track, you can get back on track and keep going.

Sounds logical, right? But how many times do you consciously remember this (and embrace it) when you find a challenge resurfacing? You've probably forgotten this wisdom as many times as I have.

If, at some point, you took some steps to change, that means you can do it again. It doesn't matter if you're taking those same steps for the second time or the seventh. Because every time you get back up and keep going, *you're assimilating the change.*

Remember, you're not the only one.

Everyone faces challenges when confronted with the need to change. No matter how enviable someone else's life looks (such as on social media), when it comes to changing, everyone faces the same challenge. Everyone has hidden resistance, no matter how it looks on the outside.

The temptation to see others as "already there" while you're still trying to figure out the game is not only

unfair to yourself, it's based on illusion. Writer and speaker Scott Stabile said it best: "After so many years struggling to keep up with you, I finally realized we're not even running the same race." Oh yeah.
Everyone is on their own unique path to change and grow.

I invite you to recall a time when you tried everything you could think of to change in a certain area of your life, but (in your own mind) you failed. Now reconsider your experience in light of the insights from this chapter. Would a better understanding of the nature of change have made a difference to your judgment that you failed? What would you do differently now? Write it in your journal so you can receive the self-affirmation you didn't get the first time.

Steps → change.
why?

Simple Tools for Change

> Synchronicity holds the promise that, if we will change within, the patterns in our outer life will change also.
> —Jean Shinoda Bolen

The points in the previous chapter were about the universal nature of change. Here are some tools for change specific to this book.

Subtle changes may begin to happen as you read.
The stories you'll be reading may stir things inside of you, such as memories or desires. The trick is to allow it. Relax and let yourself experience it.

If something important surfaces—something you sense you want to be more aware of—you'll know. That will be your cue to put the book down and consciously notice what you're feeling. But you won't need to figure anything out. You won't need to decide anything or take any action in that moment. Just allow your feelings to be seen by you.

Simply acknowledging your feelings can be powerful medicine. Acknowledging can be as uncomplicated as silently saying to a feeling, "I understand why you feel this way."

View it as getting to know yourself a little better. Even this can help inner shifts happen.

Facilitating change.
You may not notice much happening as you're reading, but your inner self will be working in the background. Change doesn't have to be a Hollywood-style transformation. Some of the most lasting change may be very subtle because it's coming from within—rather than you trying to impose it upon yourself. Instead of forcing it, you can facilitate change as you read this book by setting an intention, such as the one suggested earlier: *I'd like to discover more about myself as I read.*

Questions and invitations.
My Before & After stories will help you see yourself in the mirror. It can trigger your own discovery process in a way that doesn't need to involve self-blame—because the stories are about me, not you.

But wait a minute. Why will this be different from reading novels or watching movies? If my theory about stories is correct, shouldn't all *those* stories have changed you by now?

That's where your own participation comes in.

Most of the chapters in the rest of the book end with a few relevant questions, or an invitation to try a simple activity. The questions will help you explore your inner world. Questions can tap into deep or even hidden places, bringing you new insights about yourself.

Here's a tip for best results with the questions: thinking about it only goes so far. Writing is one of the most profound ways to access realizations that can surface from the core of your being. You can write your responses to the questions in a journal or notebook. If you don't like to write, consider doing some voice journaling using a recording app on your phone.

Quotes can help you zero in on what's vital.
A good quote is something you resonate with when it perfectly nails how you feel or think. Or a quote can show you life from someone else's perspective. Quotes are a favorite way for many people (myself included) to grasp a profound issue.

For all of these reasons, I've used pertinent quotes at the beginning of each chapter.

The remainder of this book is divided into four sections. Each section also starts with a quote, specially selected to help you get into the right frame of mind for that particular section.

If you glean some value from journaling with the questions at the ends of the chapters, you may want to journal with some of the quotes, too. But keep your heart happy and don't try to do it like "homework" (you know, where your inner adult says, "If you're going to do one, you'd better do them all!"). Simply journal about the quotes that call to you the loudest.

Reviewing this book from time to time will help you reinforce the inner changes.
If you have the paperback edition, just pick it up, let it fall open to a page, and then start reading. Oftentimes, it will be just the reminder you need.

If you're reading this book on a device, go to the table of contents and click on the first chapter title that grabs your attention. Your intuition will probably guide you to the right place.

* * *

Now that you've witnessed the story of my heart attack—and the lifestyle I regretfully lost—you probably understand why I wanted to find a way to answer my own question: *My heart attack saved my life . . . but for what?*

I've answered this in my own way, but everyone is different. By the end of the book, you'll be more aware of what your own life means to you, in ways that only you can feel and express.

In the stories that follow, I've revealed my joys and vulnerabilities, some of my best and worst memories, and my flaws and strengths. It was both scary and exhilarating. I wrote this book so I could leave a legacy—and because I'm a storyteller at heart.

> The purpose of a storyteller is not to tell you how to think, but to give you questions to think upon.
> —Brandon Sanderson

PART THREE

HEY, I'M LEARNING

The only way that we can live is if we grow.
The only way that we can grow is if we change.
The only way that we can change is if we learn.
—C. JoyBell C.

Losing Heart

> We have all been hurt. We have all had to learn painful lessons. We are all recovering from some mistake, loss, betrayal, abuse, injustice or misfortune.
> —Bryant McGill

I remember the first time I received an injection of high self-esteem. I was an eight-year-old tomboy, wearing my favorite red cowboy boots and rolled-up blue jeans. I adored my daddy and liked nothing more than to go anywhere with him.

Sometimes we'd ride in the truck to his jobsite, where his eight-man crew was busy custom-building a house. I loved to ride high up in the cab of his Ford pickup. It smelled like musty upholstery, leather, metal, and a little oil. Inhaling this perfume of Daddy, I was in heaven.

When we arrived, I'd get a special greeting from Shorty and Bill, Gilbert the cabinet maker, and Smitty, the foreman.

I must have been a sight as I jumped down from the cab, with my knotted and unbrushed platinum-white hair, little red cowboy boots, and those too-big jeans rolled at the cuffs three times. Mom would have been disappointed knowing that my hair wasn't smooth and pretty. I didn't care. I just got out of bed and went with Dad!

Sometime in the spring, Dad always went to see Grandma and Grandpa and check on the farm. Daddy co-owned the farm with his dad, and he did his share by driving two-and-a-half hours to Smith Center every few weeks.

Grandma and Grandpa lived in the best house. It was filled with shelves of Grandpa's books. Grandma's ceramic figurines were displayed in a glass case under the chiming clock. A big mirror over the fireplace reflected the front yard, with its leafy green maple trees, and the sidewalk where I could roller skate.

I loved lounging on Grandma's couch with its soft and shiny tan fabric. It was huge. I could stretch out and still only touch the midline of the long cushions. I'd pretend to be asleep so I could listen to the grown-ups talking or hear the baseball game on the fuzzy TV. Daddy and Grandpa would watch the game or talk softly about whether to plant milo or wheat in the south field.

I liked the way my cheek felt nestled into that silky fabric. Sometimes, while pretending, I would actually fall asleep.

It was in these moments that I felt so happy, content, and loved. I was like an only child, with no adorable little sisters. No sisters to compete for the attention of Mommy and Daddy.

Grandma Gracie wore an apron with big circle pockets. She called my daddy "Son." They had a brown iron pump handle in the kitchen sink. It was the first place Daddy would go after we walked in their front door.

He'd reach for a glass in the cupboard (always a jelly jar) and then pump the handle, fill the glass, and drink it straight down.

"Now that's real water! The best."

Grandma made fried chicken and cherry pies, and she let me help her. We would hang the wet laundry while the pie was baking. Grandma carried the big wicker basket, and I carried the clothespins. I would hand them to her, and she would reach up to pin them in place. I loved those moments with her in the backyard, smelling the wet sheets, and watching kids play ball in the far distance. Later, I learned that Grandpa bought the lot behind his house so he could carve out a ball field for the neighbor kids.

When night fell, Grandma cleared the supper dishes and made room for the men to play their evening game. The "men" consisted of Daddy, my Grandpa Emmett, Uncle Irwin smoking his pipe, and another uncle whose name I don't remember.

A big, flat box of dominoes was produced. Uncle Irwin would dump out the black tiles with a thunderous clatter and begin to spread them around the table facedown. I was mesmerized by those big hands shuffling the dominoes.

The men each drew eight dominoes and placed them in a semicircle with their backs facing the table. I sat at Daddy's knee and watched. The play consisted of long rows of dominoes crisscrossing the table. I quickly caught on, recognizing that the total number of white dots on the exposed ends of the dominoes had to be divisible by five.

One night, Uncle Irwin got up from the table. "Watch my hand, will you?" he said, looking at me.

My eyes were glued to the tiles. My brain was busy adding up the dots at the end of each arm. *Twelve plus twelve equals twenty-four plus sixteen equals forty. Wow!*

My foot began to tap nervously on the woven rug.

I waited for Grandpa to play his domino. My turn was next. I *knew* my move. I picked up my tile of choice, holding it between my thumb and forefinger. I made a "click click click" sound as I tapped it on Grandma's shiny oak table.

On the exposed ends sat an eight, a six, and a four. On the farthest end was the double twelve, the most valuable domino in the box. Grandpa laid down his tile at the exposed six. It was a six with one pip (one dot) on the other end. He seemed glad to be rid of it.

I took a deep breath, raised my hand, and moved it into position over the arms sprawling every which way across the table. I hovered over the exposed eight. With a slight lift to my pinky and a soft "kerplunk," I purposely laid down the double eight. Like the letter T, it lined up perpendicular.

As I scanned my hand, I smiled smugly—it was filled with eights! I knew I could play them on all the ends of my double eight.

In my most grown-up voice, I announced my total score: "45."

Uncle Irwin came back to his seat.

"What?!" He looked twice. "Why, I'll be darned, little girl. You're just as smart as these old guys around the table here!"

I peered sideways at my daddy. He was beaming.

I was so overjoyed I could barely sleep that night. I'd played a grown-up game that was rife with math problems and did it well. I did great! I was smart. Just as smart as the uncles. Just as smart as the men.

Uncle Irwin's pronouncement that night stuck with me, and I became the "smart one" in my family. I grabbed the ball and ran with it. Now I had the right to lord it over my two sisters.

* * *

During my teen years, I felt that same type of elation several more times: once when I was elected secretary of my freshman class in junior high, and again when I won the essay contest in my sophomore English class. Becoming a North High cheerleader was also exhilarating.

But the best was when I was eighteen and a senior. That year, I realized I had it made. Good grades, cheerleader, plenty of friends—and I was crowned Tower Queen of the annual River Festival.

Our classes, clubs, and teams decorated the floats for the festival. Each was adorned with flowers, crêpe paper, and scenes from student life. Each float was secured atop two canoes. Students paddled the massive display along the Little Arkansas River, which was adjacent to the high school.

A special float had been built, complete with thrones. As king and queen, we wore our robes and crowns. As royalty, we led the parade of floats. I cradled a bouquet of roses and gave the beauty queen wave, raising my hand and twisting my wrist from left to right. As each float sailed past, spectators on the riverbank cheered.

Tower Queen was different from Prom Queen or Homecoming Queen. Tower King and Queen were selected from three finalists who qualified by making average A grades. The entire school voted. I knew it was a special honor.

My self-esteem was soaring. I hummed the John Denver song "Rocky Mountain High."

• • •

He had the chiseled good looks of a young Marlon Brando or Elvis Presley, and he went to another high school.

Dating Nick suited me just fine. I loved the setup. It was cool to know I had a boyfriend who wasn't in evidence—leaving me free to roam the halls of my school without some boy hanging his arm around me, showing off his pride. I had a crush on two other boys. I had no worries and plenty of time to flirt without being interrupted. I felt free as a bird.

Nick and I would go out after Friday night football games. We'd meet somewhere at a bar to drink beer and dance. The drinking age in Kansas in the 1960s was 18. There weren't many places we could get in because Nick was only 17, but in Wichita there were neighborhood bars with a reputation for not checking ID. Because Nick was such a drinker, he and his buddies knew all these places.

Afterward, he would take me to a closed and darkened public swimming pool, to which he had the keys.

He would spread out a beach towel on the concrete floor of the dressing room. The sex was terrible. Not that I knew what to do or expect, but I never felt it to be complete. Just so much fumbling.

The stench of chlorine and shower stalls still makes me gag.

Nick had a reputation for drinking and fighting. Because we didn't go to the same school, I didn't interact with him each day, which is probably why I didn't know the real Nick.

Fall came, and I took off for Manhattan, Kansas, home of Kansas State University, my father's alma mater. I had committed to go there in eighth grade, pleasing my daddy immensely. Nick went to Emporia State College, and we would see each other some weekends.

It was one of those weekends when I got pregnant.

• • •

He was angry. Somehow it was my fault.

By today's standards, he was irresponsible, and I should have insisted on condoms. Birth control pills were not available to unmarried women in 1965.

All I knew was this: I was in trouble, and he should do the right thing.

He was 17 when we married, and he felt his future was ruined. He was mad at me the entire pregnancy, accusing me of having sex with someone else and pinning it on him.

When our son Tim was born, and in all his baby pictures, he looked just like his daddy. Nick dropped the "not mine" argument.

But there was always something disrupting our lives. We were poor, he barely made enough to pay the rent, and we had to borrow from our parents.

Nick would say mean things and treat me with disrespect. This drained every ounce of self-esteem I had once reveled in. I didn't know the words "emotional abuse," but that's what was happening.

One day, after realizing I couldn't go to the store because I had no car and no money, I began to cry. I couldn't even put a dollar together from the change I found behind the cushions. I thought of turning in bottles at the grocery store.

Instead, I walked to the riverbank near our house and sat down hard. I looked out over the same river I had been queen of a few months before. My pregnant belly was making my regular clothes too tight, so I made a maternity top using ugly brown calico fabric. I looked ridiculous.

Tears ran hot on my cheeks. I always thought that when you married a man, he would love you and take care of you and treat you like a queen. He would behave the way the only man I'd witnessed in the role of husband behaved—my daddy.

This man, this Nick, was no such thing. He was a stranger, and a mean, angry one at that.

I tried to think how I could get out of this mess. No ideas came. Just the harsh reality of my swollen belly rubbing against that stupid blouse.

Filling the Half-Empty Glass

> I, not events, have the power to make me happy or unhappy today. I can choose which it shall be. Yesterday is dead, tomorrow hasn't arrived yet. I have just one day, today, and I'm going to be happy in it.
> —Groucho Marx

Growing up in the 1950s, I knew my dad was an optimist. He was even a member of a club by the name of Optimist International. Many of his friends were members too.

The local chapter met at a nearby restaurant for lunch meetings every Friday. Besides the lunch meetings, they raised funds for scholarships with their annual Christmas tree lot. Mom joined the Opti-Mrs. Club, the group for spouses of members. The women raised funds with book drives and fashion shows.

As a young adult, Daddy would take me along to lunch meetings. I liked it because I got to be with my dad, have a free lunch, and eavesdrop on adult conversation.

My dad passed away in the 1980s. The one thing I claimed as my own from his home office was the plaque with the "Optimist Creed." Years later, when I read the words on the plaque, I knew where our family got its "glass half-full" attitude.

> *The Optimist Creed*
>
> *Promise yourself to be SO STRONG that nothing can disturb your peace of mind. To talk health, happiness, and prosperity to every person you meet. To make all your friends feel that there is something in them.*

I remember the dramatic impact of the words the members said in unison at every meeting. The president would announce the closing of the meeting. That was the cue for everyone in the room to stand and shout in their loudest voice, "Man! Do I feel good!"

As part of the ritual, the men performed a synchronized movement: clenching the right fist, bending the right elbow, and then—at the exact moment of the shout—plunging the fist down and to the left.

"Man! Do I feel good!"

Everyone who walked out of that meeting had the most wonderful afternoon.

• • •

As a kid, my glass was always half-full.

My optimistic life view stayed with me until darkness hit in 1965. I found myself thrown into a grown-up role I knew nothing about. I was 18, married to an angry man-boy, and pregnant with a baby coming in a few short months. All I really wanted was my college experience with my classmates at Kansas State University.

My mind was a writhing mass of worries. My heart was hurting from all the negative thoughts boiling in my head. Each resulting negative feeling brought stinging tears. I was filled with guilt, remorse, sadness, and failure.

It was the first time in my life that I felt so low.

My glass had drained, and now it was less than half-empty. I couldn't see one positive glimmer on my horizon. My thinking switched from positive to negative overnight.

Living paycheck to paycheck, with no car, alone all day and pregnant, my life was a blur. I had endless hours to kill. For something to do, I'd watch the old boxy TV with the foil-wrapped antennae, but soap operas didn't even begin to fill the void.

After Timmy was born, I finally had a source of pleasure. I could pick him up, cuddle him, change him, nurse him, and "play." He was a miracle, and I had fun adoring him.

One piece of advice to young mothers is to sleep when the baby sleeps. However, like many new mothers, I saw those few hours of baby-quiet as a chance to get the chores done.

I had inherited my grandma's pink Maytag. My mom's machine, the one I'd seen her use a million times, was top-loading. This Maytag front-loader was a mystery. After stuffing the clothes in and adding detergent, I would close the door with its special lock. As it churned, I could watch it like a television screen.

One time, I was washing diapers and wanted to add bleach. What to do? The window showed sudsy water sloshing around with the clothes. I took a deep breath, turned the knob to stop between cycles, poured a cup of liquid bleach, opened the door, and tossed it in. Water sloshed on the floor.

Oh, my. All the things I didn't know.

The load finished with a final spin. I opened the door to a strong aroma of bleach and pulled the wet things into a big wicker basket. Hefting the basket onto my hip, I trudged out the back door to the clothesline.

As I hung the diapers, the air began to chill. I realized I should have hung these out in the morning so the warm afternoon sun would help them dry faster.

After that chore was done, the baby woke up. I changed and fed him. Nick came home from work, and I set the table for dinner. We were done early, just as the sun was setting. I had completely forgotten about those diapers on the line.

It rained that night. I was learning the hard way about keeping house. I didn't like it. I longed to be on the college campus with my friends in Manhattan.

I desperately wanted a life. My days were filled with taking care of my sweet baby, cleaning the three rooms of our house, and wondering what would become of me.

I wanted to feel stimulated and engaged. Instead, I was in a perpetual fog. I wanted my brain to wake up! I didn't have any books to read, and my magazines were tattered from reading them so often.

I thought and thought.

How can I feel better?

My mind wouldn't stop asking the same question.

• • •

By the time Tim was born I was 19½ years old. All the girls I'd gone to high school with now had that 1960s cute college girl image that I'd wanted for myself. I couldn't wait to get my regular body shape back.

At 20, I couldn't wait any longer to find my path. I had little experience to draw from—but I did remember feeling smart and stimulated during my school years. Maybe going back to school would be the best thing for me.

The more I thought about it, the more it seemed right. I remembered my younger years at Garrison Elementary, where I was rewarded and praised for doing well and being smart. I loved the feeling of receiving extra credit from one of my favorite teachers just for doing something I loved.

Junior high and high school gave me plenty of opportunities to shine academically, which boosted my confidence even more.

My intuition kept telling me something that excited me: if I continued my education, my mind would remember feeling positive.

I prayed, I talked to myself, and I ran through scenarios in my mind. Finally, I came to a decision. I decided no one could get me out of this sucking sinkhole but me.

• • •

During the 1960s, a young lady's career path consisted of two options: become a teacher or become a nurse. I knew I didn't want either for my future.

I laid out a plan to get a degree in subjects I knew would be fulfilling: fashion merchandising and interior design. Those were my dream careers.

My sisters and I had a college fund to cover our education expenses. I know we were privileged, but I had counted on a wonderful time having a college experience. So much for that golden plan.

Instead, on a sunny Wednesday morning, I dialed the number for the private school.

• • •

Patricia Stevens Career College and Modeling School was in downtown Wichita. I met with the manager, Mrs. Moeder, and she gave me a tour of the school. An elegantly appointed lobby, management offices, and a spacious meeting room took up the ground floor. The classrooms, a makeup studio, and a gym with a wall of mirrors were upstairs.

The fold-out color brochure showed smiling young women working in clothing stores, surrounded by beautiful gowns and dresses. One panel featured a brunette displaying fabric samples to a design client. Open that panel and there were pretty girls modeling on a runway, arm in arm, bowing to the audience.

Inside the brochure, I saw the courses and specialties being offered. The courses sounded interesting and fun. As a bonus, there was the modeling training, which might come in handy at some point.

The degree issued by the school was one of the selling points. The degree would outline the skills acquired to qualify for a job in fashion merchandising, interior design, or fashion modeling. I was happy to read that all this education, the fascinating courses, and the modeling training could be completed in nine months.

There was even a bonus. At the end of your studies, the school would place you with an employer in your chosen field.

It was a fast-track, complete education, but it was not cheap. I would need money from my college fund, but this meant I could get the education I wanted. Then I could use my smarts to get into the workforce pronto.

I asked my parents for the balance of my college fund, paid the tuition, and set up a savings account to pay a babysitter. I bought two dresses, a coat, a silk scarf, and a pair of low-heel pumps. I hadn't had any new clothes since my college wardrobe.

* * *

Classes were held Monday through Thursday, from eight o'clock to noon.

I started learning new things right away. The first classes were geared toward the modeling curriculum. Our instructor was a professional model. Six of us sat at lighted, oval-shaped mirrors and learned to apply basic makeup for modeling.

We practiced walking up and down stairs without looking down or turning our heads. We spent an hour in the mirrored gym, each student walking with a book on her head. We even took fencing lessons to build confidence and sportsmanship.

Later, we had classes for merchandising and marketing products. I was like a sponge, learning something new every day.

The best part was when Mrs. Arlene Van Zandt came to teach interior design. She was a statuesque woman with silver hair and silver jewelry, and she owned her own design studio.

Mrs. Van Zandt set up a display made from bolts of fabric. There were intricate damasks, velvets, and woven blends for upholstery. For drapes and curtains, there were chiffons, slubbed satins, and patterned cottons.

In this fun class, I also had access to *The History of Furniture: Twenty-Five Centuries of Style and Design in the Western Tradition*. Poring over glossy photos of beautiful pieces from the Renaissance period, sturdy, functional designs from the 1930s, and so much more, I was in heaven.

Mr. Phillips came another day. He was nearly bald and wore wire-rim glasses. He was the manager of Alliance Interiors, an interior design showroom downtown. He brought carpet samples and talked to us about durability, carpet wear, loops, and cut pile.

I ran my hand over my favorite sample.

"It's the latest trend," he said. "Shag carpet. You keep it looking new with a plastic rake."

I couldn't wait to go to the showroom to see an entire room carpeted in shag.

One day the school announced that any of us could volunteer for a haircut by the Vidal Sassoon team from London. You'd have to be of a certain age to know who Vidal Sassoon was—the most famous hairdresser of the 1960s, creating styles that boosted women's sense of personal freedom. Some say he changed the craft of hairstyling forever.

I volunteered and got his signature cut: a short bob, with one side shorter over the ear. It was angular, modern, and felt so liberating.

• • •

One month before graduation, Mrs. Moeder took me aside.

"Susan, I've arranged an interview for you with one of Wichita's most prestigious interior designers."

I couldn't believe my good fortune.

The following week, I borrowed my mother's Lincoln Continental to drive to my interview. I had an appointment with John Palous, owner and founder of the interior design studio.

Palous wore baggy pants, a Guayabera shirt, and loafers with no socks. His office had two rooms, one with a massive desk and one with a huge worktable strewn with blueprints, room sketches, and watercolor images of clients' rooms.

I adored the quaint, converted Victorian house with its brick paver courtyard. The big windows facing the front showcased a beautiful gift shop, filled with Waterford crystal and silver décor items. These pieces would end up in the most beautiful homes in Wichita.

I got the job! Part-time in the afternoons, after my morning classes. I typed and mailed invoices, and did typing work for the in-house architect. In my role of secretary-receptionist, I would greet clients and take them through a gallery-like hallway to John's office.

The bar in John's office was stocked with Bombay Gin and Johnnie Walker Scotch Whisky. Customers would mingle at lunchtime, and John would play bartender, mixing generous drinks in squat crystal highball glasses. It was so casual there, not like any workplace I'd known of or seen on TV.

I fell in love with the quirky staff. I went to the furniture market in Dallas with junior designers Deanne and Larry. I even went on some of the jobs with John's designers, carrying sample books for fabrics and carpet.

I was given more responsibility. I got a raise. The business grew. I loved that job. I was happy.

I invite you to think of a time when you created your own turnaround, even though things seemed hopeless. How did you recapture your happiness? If it was about following your heart, how exactly did you do that? Having a written record of it in your journal could be priceless.

The Power of Choice

Life is a matter of choices, and every choice you make MAKES YOU.
—John Maxwell

By the time I was 27, I had lived a long, hard, and lesson-filled existence.

One Easter weekend, Nick was caught and arrested in an assault case involving a young woman. The first cop on the scene happened to be a friend, who got him out of trouble as quickly as he got into it. But that was it! I'd waited for him to do something so terrible that no one would blame me for leaving him.

It worked. His parents shipped him off to an AA camp to dry out, and then to an uncle's home to attend college.

After divorcing Nick and getting on with my life, I thought I had finally turned the corner. I believed I'd found the answers to all my problems. Prince Charming swept in to save the day, and I moved from Kansas (the home of my problems) to Arizona (the home of the man of my dreams).

This time around, it was a man with money who loved me and wanted to take care of me and my two little boys, Timmy and Nathan. I was so happy to get out of that hard life, and to finally have money, and the chance to live my life without worry.

I did everything to please him. I was anxious to accomplish our shared goals. One was to retire at 40, manage our investments, and travel the world. By the time we grownups hit our dream goal of becoming millionaires, my boys would be finished with school.

I didn't have to work. My new husband made that clear. Not having to work was a treat—no more arranging babysitters or daycare for the kids. This was a big change for me.

Ron bought a sweet, burnt-adobe brick home on Tucson's Eastside. What a nice neighborhood, I thought. Our house even had a pool!

"Every house in Tucson has a swimming pool," Ron informed me. "No big deal."

It was nothing like the ranch-style homes with the rambling green lawns and long, curving driveways I had known in Kansas. This house had a yard of gravel and large rocks.

"It's called desert landscaping," Ron said. "All the houses have it."

I had a lot to get used to in this foreign land.

* * *

Walking the two blocks to the neighborhood school, Brown Elementary, I was distracted. Ron's voice was loud in my mind, sharing with me his nightly recital of hopes and dreams.

"I'm thinking about adopting the boys. That way they'll have the same last name as me."

He paused before adding the grand finale.

"I'm waiting for *Success Magazine* to call and book a photo shoot. I want to include you and the kids."

I couldn't stop thinking about that photo: Mr. Successful Businessman with his lovely wife and children, smiling out from the glossy pages.

Nathan was holding my hand while taking giant strides to avoid stepping on sidewalk cracks.

"What did you think of Ron's idea? You know, about adoption? And changing your last name?"

Silence. He dipped his head.

"How about you, Tim?"

Tim's eyes slanted as he glared at me. "Do I have to?"

"No, of course not," I said. "It will just make everything easier—getting you enrolled in school and after-school sports."

More silence.

"We don't have to talk about it right now. Let's go inside. Maybe they'll have advanced classes like you had before we moved."

"Hope so."

In the office, a chipper, gray-haired woman with pink glasses greeted us at a wooden counter. I enrolled Tim in the third grade.

"Is there a GATE program here?" I asked.

GATE stands for Gifted and Talented Education.

Tim piped up. "I was in it last year at my other school."

"Why, yes," the nice office lady said. "We do have a similar program. They do the testing at the beginning of the school year. This school year will be over in two months, so he can test next year."

Tim was looking at the bright posters covering the wall, featuring art by students of different grades. Mrs. Gray Hair noticed his interest.

"That bright blue poster is your class. Your teacher is Ms. Littleton."

He wandered closer for a better look.

Ms. Gray Hair leaned forward and peered down over the counter. "What about this one?" she said, looking at Nathan. "How old are you, young man?"

Nathan clung to my skirt and peered up at me. He shyly held up four fingers.

"When is his birthday?"

"The third of October," I stammered. "He's not old enough to enroll. Is he?"

I heard Ron talking in my head. "Wouldn't that be great? Both kids in school! That would make life easier." His voice, as usual, was convincing.

I realized I hadn't been listening. I snapped to it and paid attention. "In Arizona, the cutoff dates are different. He's eligible as long as his birthday is before the last day of December."

She smiled and pushed her glasses farther up her nose.

"He can start school next week when his brother does. He will have Ms. Byers for kindergarten."

My mind was whirling. I hadn't planned on both kids going to school next week.

Ron's voice was chattering with excitement. "Go ahead! Make it happen. Just think about it, Susan—you could go back to work or just have free time."

I smiled back at her. "Why, yes, let's do that. Where do I sign?"

* * *

Nathan struggled in school and had to repeat fourth grade.

By then, we were millionaires. We lived in a huge, mansion-like house on 20 acres, far from the school and my children's friends. My husband paid attention to Tim but not to Nathan.

Later, the teenage Nathan started missing school, staying locked in his room brooding. We started family counseling, each of us suffering from some emotional trauma.

Nathan began running away. He would stay with friends for a night or two, then call me to bring him home.

One day he didn't come back. I was sick with worry.

I had read studies showing that children, especially boys, do better in school if they start later. I thought back to the day I was so excited to get him into school, and the choice I made so I could have free time in my new life.

Nathan's downward spiral started in kindergarten and wouldn't end until he was 30.

* * *

In my late 40s, I began attending church on a regular basis. I would go by myself, sit in the back, and take notes on the sermon. I found solace in each week's message.

One Sunday, I felt a tap on my shoulder. Turning, I was shocked to see Roberta Bentley, the mother-in-law from my long-ago past. It had been nearly twenty years.

"Roberta. What are you doing here?"

Roberta looked much the same. Her watery blue eyes were paler, her hair had gone to silver, and she wore a cotton shirtwaist dress with a belt, just like always.

She twisted a hanky as she spoke. "I moved to Tucson after Jean died."

Her voice was shaky and nervous, just as I remembered.

"Well, what a surprise!" I said. "Welcome to Tucson, and welcome to our church." With that, I turned on my heel. "I have to run now. Meeting a friend for lunch. Bye."

I couldn't wait to get out of there. My heart was pounding, and a flood of emotions washed over me. I vividly remembered all the situations when her words and actions had left me feeling like a bad mother. I felt my face flush with anger and humiliation.

• • •

The next week, there she was again. She sat directly behind me. The congregation was reading the Apostles' Creed in unison when I heard her coughing.

Oh, there's nothing worse than having that tickle and a cough in church.

The thought ran silently through my mind as I remembered doing it myself, earning a few hard stares from nearby members. I opened my handbag and pawed through to the bottom.

"There it is!" I whispered.

I turned and handed a honey cough drop to my coughing ex-mother-in-law. Her watery eyes blinked as if to say, "Oh, thank you."

After the service, she stood waiting for me.

"I want to thank you for the cough drop. It really saved me."

"You're welcome," I said. "See you next week."

I watched her walk slowly into the courtyard.

My church's courtyard is a lovely spot, much like a covered patio, with a low brick wall perfect for sitting. A gentle breeze floated through, bringing the fragrance of jasmine from a vine running along one of the beams. Long banquet tables covered with white plastic tablecloths sat at each corner. One for coffee service, one with lemonade, one with water, and one in the middle piled high with cookies.

Clusters of people stood on the concrete, talking and smiling. A man held a leather-bound bible while he chatted with a couple I'd seen before. Two little girls chased each other, grabbing treats as they ran around the cookie table.

I watched Roberta pass right by Kathy Feller, who was welcoming members.

Such a lonely figure.

● ● ●

My son Tim called the next week.

"Grandma Bentley has moved to Tucson."

"I know! I saw her at church."

"I'm thinking of having a barbecue at my house for all of us. What do you think?"

I knew I had a choice to make, and not much time to think.

"Good idea. Do you think we can get Nathan to come?"

Before I knew it, a family gathering was planned, including Grandma Bentley.

"Everybody's bringing a dish," Tim reported. "She can't wait to make her famous cucumber salad and chocolate cake."

I felt an old anxiety trigger somewhere in my gut. "Great, I can't wait," I said quietly.

The day came for the potluck and cookout. I purposely came a little late. I didn't want to be part of a greeting committee. My hands were full as I pushed open the front door.

"Hi, everyone! I brought chips and dip and a veggie tray."

Tim ushered me into the kitchen. "Here, let me take those from you. Oh, and here's a glass of your favorite Chardonnay."

Oh my, he knows me well.

Sensing my anxiety and nerves, his gesture of a glass of wine was perfect.

Tim and Christina were the perfect hosts. Their house in the foothills enjoys an impressive view. Tim had seated Roberta in the dining room so she could catch the stunning mountain view.

I noticed she was wringing her hanky, and her eyes watered even more than before. I greeted her.

"What do you think of this pretty place? And Tucson in general?"

"I do like it," she answered, in that trembling voice. "Especially the church. Everyone is so friendly."

We chit-chatted about this and that. Was it the wine? I realized I was beaming. I felt happy and relaxed. Roberta was beaming, too, and finally looking relaxed.

After eating, we all sat around the table, sipping coffee and talking.

"Next time, we'll do this at my house," I said into the chatter.

Roberta smiled at me.

Consider journaling about choices in your life—both good and bad—that ended up being powerful or long-lasting. When you read back over what you wrote, can you tell whether these choices came from your head or your heart?

Multitasking My Life Away

> Every human being is the author of his own health or disease.
> —Buddha

I used to relish the challenge of a deadline—especially if it was really important and really big. I would jump into Superwoman mode and work harder, faster, smarter. I would have fun putting pressure on myself to get it done.

Maybe I was being competitive. Maybe I was showing off. Or maybe I was just feeling the thrill of risk-taking. All I know is how much I loved the adrenaline.

Multitasking was a related thrill.

"I'm a good multitasker," I'd brag to my friends. "Doing more than one thing at a time gives me energy!"

* * *

It was time to pack. Our long summer vacation in Oregon was coming up.

"I'll need all your stuff by tomorrow morning," Tomas announced.

"Sure thing!" I chirped.

Tomas planned to drive there early, check on the motorhome, unpack our stuff, and get settled.

"I'll meet you in a month," I'd said when we finalized our plans. "I have a non-stop flight picked out."

Now there was just the packing.

"This should be easy," I told myself. "It's one hundred degrees here in Tucson, and seventy in Oregon, dropping to forty at night. Anything warm and fuzzy, for sure!"

I started in the hall closet, pulling out jackets and coats and dumping them on the bed. My next trip to the hall closet had me standing on tiptoe, reaching high to grab my prize from the top shelf. I could barely see the ugly purple nylon zip-up duffle bag that I refused to throw away.

"This thing holds a lot! I'm sure I'll need it."

It slid off the shelf, hitting me on the head. A wave of dizziness washed over me. I rapidly lowered my heels so I could feel my feet on the floor.

The purple bag was slippery as it came undone from the neat fold of last summer. It slapped against my legs, almost tripping me. I dragged it slowly into the bedroom and added it to the mound on the bed.

Feeling better, I took all of my jeans out of the dresser drawer and added them to the pile. "That's way too many!" I scolded. "You'll have to try them all on."

The trying-on process uncovered new issues.

"These go better with boots, and the light-wash ones are better with tennis shoes."

I stopped to think it through.

"That reminds me. I should pack my boots and tennies and the shoes I keep for cold, wet weather."

I dropped the jeans I'd been about to try on and went to my closet to dig through the shoe bins.

"What are you doing?" Tomas said.

I jumped. I had not heard him come up behind me. Looking at my heap, he smiled in his shrewd way.

"You'll never be able to get into bed for your nap today."

"Don't worry," I said, pawing through a bottom drawer of socks. "I know what I'm doing."

"You shouldn't be bending over so much," he warned.

"I know, I know. But when I do it really fast, I barely feel it."

Tomas shook his head.

Now I had a stack of shoes and boots and a messy pile of socks on the floor of the closet. My cell phone vibrated. Glancing at the screen, I saw it was my youngest sister, Mary.

"Hi, sister!" I said, as I stood up and backed out of the cluttered closet. "Let me go into a different room," I added, glad to leave the gigantic mess behind.

"I'm looking for Robin's address. Will you send it to me?"

"Sure. How are you feeling today?"

I was worried about her. Her recent case of COVID-19 still lingered, and she was coughing.

"I'm still not 100 percent. I can't wait to feel better." She paused. "What about you? You sound out of breath. What on Earth are you doing?"

"Packing up some things for Oregon. Tomas wants to take them ahead of time so I can fly next month and not schlep everything." I paced around my office. "He gave me a packing deadline. I felt sure I could knock it out in a couple of hours. I thought it would be easy, but it's wearing me out."

"I think you should sit down and take a break. Drink some water. Okay?"

"Oh, Mary, now you sound like me. Remember, *I'm* the bossy big sister!"

I found the address Mary wanted, and we said our sisterly goodbyes.

"Now, I must get back to my packing mess."

The tower of stuff on the bed was about to tip over. The jeans I'd meant to try on lay in two rumpled piles. I thought about the warm sweaters I wanted and slowly opened the deep bottom drawer of the antique dresser. I couldn't decide which ones to take, so I gathered them all into my arms, adding them to the mountain on the bed.

"Well, at least everything is in one spot."

My cell phone rang again. "Hi, Nancy!"

"Are you okay? You sound out of breath."

"I'm fine. Just rushing around, trying to pack for Oregon."

I nudged a pile of jeans with my toe.

"Susan, did you remember that I'm coming by today? So I can pick up those boxes of greeting bags and supplies for the health fair next weekend?"

"Oh, sure." I glanced at the clock. "What time do you want to come over?"

"I'm out right now. I figure I'll be there in thirty minutes."

"Great. I'll have them ready for you."

I *had* forgotten . . . but I was pretty sure I knew right where they were.

Leaving the mountain on the bed, I walked through the messy kitchen. The countertops were littered with canned goods, boxes, and plastic grocery bags. "Oh, darn, I forgot to put the groceries away."

I stepped over a spill of salt from last night's popcorn. "I'll just sweep this up first." Slipping into the garage, I reached for the broom and its matching blue plastic dust pan. "Nobody wants to step on salt."

Sweep. Sweep. Scoop, scoop. The spilled salt was gone. I kept sweeping, eyeing a sprinkle of coffee grounds and a stray fluff of dust. Sweep. Sweep. Scoop, scoop. The lid of the garbage can banged shut.

Back in the garage, I scanned the boxes stacked floor to ceiling along both walls.

"Now, where are those boxes of volunteer supplies?"

I caught a glimpse of the distinctive, red-tagged boxes on the far wall. Of course, Tomas's truck was parked right there.

"Darn. I'll have to ask him to move it."

I summoned my breath.

"Honey?" I called. "Will you move the truck? I have to get something from that side of the garage."

When he showed up, he was sweating in the Tucson heat. "What is it now?"

"Nancy is coming over, and I promised her two boxes of supplies for the health fair."

His face was stern. "Okay. Let me get the keys."

Once the east wall was visible, I could see that one was up high, and the other was near the bottom of the pile. Standing on my tiptoes, I reached for the upper box.

"Oh, no, you don't! Let me get that for you."

Tomas easily pulled it out of the stack, setting it on the laundry table. "Is that it?"

"The other one's in the next row," I pointed. "Down by those Christmas decorations."

Grunting and tugging, he pulled the box from its wedged-in spot and placed it on the laundry table.

"Are you almost ready for me to load your packing?"

"Uh-huh," I fibbed. "Just about."

I went back to the bedroom and looked at my piles. My arms hurt from reaching up. My back hurt from bending over. And my collarbone was aching. I walked carefully to the doorway of my husband's project room. He was bending over a table of boxed-up tools.

"Honey?" I said faintly. "I need to talk to you."

He looked up, not smiling. "What's up?"

"I can't be ready as soon as I thought." My voice cracked a little. "All I've done is get everything out—but it's not packed up."

I gently rubbed my aching collarbone.

"Plus, I'm exhausted. I really need to lie down."

Before he could answer, I turned and made my way to the sofa. I propped up my feet, closed my eyes, and fell asleep.

Are you hooked on multitasking? Can you recognize when you're doing it? In your journal, record a portion of your day (even just an hour) to see if you can spot where your habits of multitasking are hidden. Awareness can help you break the habit.

Resistance Is Futile

> The pain that you create now is always some form of nonacceptance, some form of unconscious resistance to what is.
> —Eckhart Tolle

Jamie was my latest physical therapist. Because of COVID, he was wearing a black N95 mask—the type with external exhaust valves—over a traditional blue mask. I could see his brown eyes below his receding hairline and bushy eyebrows. I expected his voice to sound like Darth Vader's.

"Do this," he said, as he stood on one foot.

I tried it, immediately wobbling to my left.

"I've got you," he said, yanking the balance belt hard. "Now try it again. This time with your eyes closed."

"Do I have to?" I whined. "I never do this in real life. I mean, why would I?"

I was doing physical therapy to improve my strength and regain my sense of balance. I vividly remembered Dr. Sarah's words: "Loss of balance is just one thing a stroke does to your brain." Oh, great. I was learning the hard way that even a mini-stroke can have a substantial impact.

During the previous 12 months, I'd been to three PT facilities, each with a different therapist. Highly trained and good-hearted, they each came up with torturous exercises.

"It's for your own good."

They could sing that line in a choir of therapists, I thought bitterly.

Later in the session, I waited while Jamie put the finishing touches on a complex obstacle course: orange cones, three square foam cushions, and a series of hard plastic steps.

"Oh, no!" I moaned. "I hate those squishy cushions, especially when you make me stand on them and close my eyes."

I made my way through the course, wavering with every step. As I tried to steady myself on top of two three-inch cushions, I froze.

"I feel like I'm on top of the Empire State Building."

Finally, I gingerly lifted my knee and quickly set my foot down firmly on the floor.

"Now do it again sideways."

Jamie laughed as he spoke. I scrunched up my eyes and glared at him.

"Ha. I knew I could get *that* look from you today!"

He sounded way too gleeful for my liking.

I glanced at the wall clock. Oh, goodie, our time was almost up. Jamie took a 10-pound weighted pipe and stretched it out in front of him.

"Now you try it. Hold your arms out straight." He demonstrated like a gymnast. "Now raise it over your head, and then pull it down to your thighs."

I was determined to do it, but it was so hard.

"This is making me nauseous! And I'll never do this in real life!"

I wanted to go home.

The following week, Jamie had me walking backwards.

"This scares me. I can't sense where I'm stepping."

He nodded emphatically.

"That's the whole point. You need to remember how to walk backwards."

"No, I don't! I swear I never step backwards in my daily life. Why don't we work on something else?"

He had reduced me to my begging voice again, and I hated it.

"Trust me. This *is* a part of your life." I could almost hear Jamie grinning behind his mask.

"But, but. . . ." I sputtered. I was out of arguments.

• • •

I walked into Target with my daughter-in-law, Melissa. "We'll do some back-to-school shopping," I said, as I grasped the cart handle. Having the cart to hold on to gave me confidence.

After we'd been up and down a few aisles, I felt the call of nature. Darn.

"I need to go to the restroom. I'll be right back."

"Do you need me to go with you?" Melissa asked.

"No. It's just over there, by the door. And, besides, I have the cart to hold on to."

The restroom was spacious, with white, diamond-shaped tiles on the floor. I chose the handicap stall at the end. I like those. They have grab bars. The stall door was extra wide and opened outward for wheelchair access. As I reached to close the door, a realization hit me.

I would have to step backwards.

I faced the door. Tentatively placing my right foot one step back, I held on to the tiny door handle with all my might. Closing my eyes, I put my left foot back, trying to calm my fear of falling. Long seconds ticked by as I shuffled in slow, backwards steps.

I was finally able to pull that damn door shut.

By now, I was perspiring and had to stop for breath. Jamie's masked face flashed before me.

"Oh, crap," I said to the door.

Recall a time when you were asked (or told) to do something that was good for you or meant to help you in life. How did you react? If you experienced resistance, what sparked it? Journaling honestly about your resistance behaviors can help you understand yourself and your feelings more deeply, bringing in compassion.

Control vs. Flow

> May what I do flow from me like a river, no forcing and no holding back, the way it is with children.
> —Rainer Maria Rilke

When I was 10, Mrs. Hurst was teaching fourth and fifth grade in the same classroom. Often, I finished the assignments early, and she would invite me to work on a craft project.

In November, she asked me to create a mural on the back wall of the classroom. The wall was about nine feet across and covered with cork, making a huge bulletin board. She told me I could decide what the mural would be. When I heard this, my imagination raced.

I had seen the first animated Disney movie, *Cinderella*. I was entranced by the pumpkin turning into a coach pulled by mice, and infatuated with the handsome Prince Charming. Somehow, my mind came around to combining pumpkins and Thanksgiving and the Cinderella story.

I started cutting construction paper pumpkins, mice, characters, and scenery. As I created the shapes, I used thumbtacks to secure them to the cork board. I decided to make the characters move, so I detached the arms and legs and then used gold brads to secure their limbs back onto their bodies.

I was in a dream world, cutting construction paper freehand and reveling in the colors—oranges, browns, and greens for the season, vibrant blue for Cinderella's dress, and deep red for Prince Charming's cloak. I especially loved the adorable mice. But the pinnacle of my joy was the pumpkin coach, complete with moving wheels.

I spent three days creating my masterpiece. I stretched up high to put Prince Charming's hat with its feather plume into position. Nobody broke the spell I was in.

Finally, it was complete. Kids gathered around, smiling and clapping. Teachers stopped by to see the mammoth Cinderella mural on Mrs. Hurst's classroom wall. It was like no other room decoration in the history of our school.

* * *

Back when I used to create jewelry, I would often find myself "in the flow."

Whenever I got quite far along stringing beads, crystals, and stones on a slim wire, I would clip it closed and lay it on a soft white cloth. This would allow me to tell whether the design was appealing.

I loved this part of the process, playing with colors and textures to see which ones worked best. I built a design table where I did nothing but lay out beads and explore the many combinations. Sometimes I would sketch them in my design notebook. The reverie I felt was heartwarming.

During the 1970s, I took on sewing and dressmaking to make some extra money. I splurged and purchased a Bernina sewing machine, paying $45 a month until it was paid off. That machine ran like a dream, whether it was stitching a seam at top speed, or easing in a curved shoulder seam, slow and steady.

My next purchase was a pair of electric scissors. I could cut fabric in seconds! I was really in the flow.

Janet, a graceful, slim brunette, asked me to make her some custom clothing. She would purchase a complex Vogue pattern, and the softest wool jersey, fine denier wool gabardine, or luxurious silk. This gave me the opportunity to touch and work with fine fabrics, while putting together those complex Vogue designs. It was heavenly.

I also loved my years spent working in retail clothing. I worked in ladies' stores, boutiques, and department stores. I did everything: store manager, buyer, and advertising manager. I even had my own store.

My favorite part was stocking the store when new clothes arrived. I'd cut open the boxes, shake out the folded clothes, put a hanger through the neck and shoulders, and run my fingers down the side of the garment.

I'd slip the hook of the hanger over the smooth metal bar on the rolling rack. Then another and another, until the new stock was ready to roll out onto the floor. There, I would ask a floor manager to help me hang the new pieces.

I'd fall into a trance-like rhythm, clicking the hangers from the rolling rack onto the double-rod display rack on the sales floor. Once I was satisfied with the order of the clothes on the rack, I'd slip my hand between the styles and push the garments to one side. *Swoosh* went the metal hangers on the shiny rod. This always made me smile.

• • •

During my 18 years of being single, I entered a season in my life where I was tired of running around, dating guys here and there, and feeling left out of couples' events.

I knew Bobby from around town. His business was a video and marketing company. He was creative and had a talent for capturing a person's essence on film. These became local commercials. Some were classics.

The more we crossed paths, the more I noticed sparks.

I was asked to make a video promoting a local golf tournament with national sponsors. I set up the filming appointments, and Bobby crafted the final edited commercial. I was fascinated with his studio, sound-board, and equipment. It was magical watching him set the visual moments to music. He seemed to know every song from every era.

No one could guess his age. Tall, slim, and handsome, Bobby had a swagger to his walk and a slight lean when he was still. You could swear James Dean was in the room, complete with the slouch, the relaxed cigarette, and the falling lock of hair.

His youthful charm was irresistible in small doses but silly and immature in large doses. I was in the small-dose category. I found him charming and witty, and he was a great dancer. Oh, and he could sing.

After we started dating, any time we went somewhere that had live music, Bobby would take to the stage and sing a perfect impression of Elvis or Dean Martin. It was always a beautiful love song to me. The audience ate it up, cheering him every time.

I loved our dates, riding in a little Volkswagen convertible, music blasting, hitting the fun nightspots. We were inseparable.

He asked me to move in with him, promising he could make his little cracker-box house work for me, a woman with unusual closet needs. Whenever I looked for apartments, I always looked for ways to accomplish the 48 feet of closet rod space I knew I would need.

Bobby pulled a folded piece of paper from his wallet. "Look what I designed." I saw lines, squares attached by dotted lines, and more lines. "I'm going to build onto the house."

I knew I didn't want that. I wasn't crazy about the small house and its overgrown yard. Plus, the neighborhood was sketchy. After a moment's thought, I said, "Why not move into my place until you get the construction figured out?"

The next day was a crisp, sunny fall day. I drove my red Honda Prelude to the little house. Pushing on the front door, I could walk right in.

Boldly, I went to the tiny closet in his tiny bedroom. I pulled out all the shirts, pants, and jackets and laid them on the bed. Then I put as many in my car as would fit.

Back at my condo, I hauled all the clothes into the guest room and hung them in the spacious closet.

On my next trip to his place, I emptied the drawers of his miniature dresser. Everything fit perfectly in the dresser in my guest room.

He was at work that day and didn't have a clue what I was doing. Later, when he expressed shock, I defended my actions.

"I thought you'd be happy! I saved you some work and moved your clothes in for you."

Christmas came.

"Let's order everything from these catalogs and have them shipped," I said excitedly.

He was quiet. "Sure, I guess so."

"We're going to Houston for Christmas," I announced. "We can stay at my sister's."

"Sure, I guess so," he said. "We'll celebrate with my mom and Eric beforehand?"

I had forgotten about them, but I said, "Sure."

The Houston trip was telling. I realized Bobby had never experienced a fun-loving, functional family like mine. His father left his mother when he was a baby, and he had a 10-year-old son with his estranged wife. I watched in disbelief as he made himself at home with the little kids, the pets, and my sisters. It was clear he knew nothing about boundaries.

One day, a red fire engine drove through the subdivision, its siren blaring. All the kids ran outside. Of course, Bobby did too.

"Santa was on the fire engine!" he said, out of breath from running down the street. I wished he wouldn't act so childish.

The following month, he asked me to marry him. I said no immediately. I knew I didn't want to marry him and felt I was falling out of love with him.

"I've done everything your way since the day you moved my clothes in," Bobby said. "I thought you loved me and wanted to get married. But now I think you just like controlling our relationship."

"Hmm?" I thought.

We went to a friend's wedding. Bobby had to sit down several times, complaining of dizziness. The next day, he fainted. His headaches were severe.

I took time off work to take him to the ER, where they performed an MRI.

"It's a tumor the size of a baseball," they said.

The cancer whirlwind began. Surgery was scheduled first, then radiation after that. Bobby's treatment was new and experimental. His case was unique. His oncologist was even interviewed by the media.

"What am I going to do?" I wailed to my best friend.

"Get out now," she said. "This cancer could make you a caregiver for the rest of your life. And you're not even sure you love him!"

As much as her words pained me, I knew she was right. I couldn't give Bobby the love and care he would need to get through this battle. Despite her well-meaning advice, I stayed. Because who leaves a man newly diagnosed with brain cancer and no one to take care of him?

Even though my job was new, I had the flexibility to run back and forth to the hospital. The surgery was gruesome, cutting open his scalp, then cutting a piece of his skull in a rectangular shape and removing it to get at the giant tumor.

"It's in the frontal lobe, so I'm hoping we can get it all," reported Mr. Famous Brain Surgeon. "If not, the radiation will take care of the rest."

Bobby was a good sport and a good patient. I don't remember how his medical bills were paid, but he never spoke of it.

He stayed in the hospital for radiation treatment. It was a one-shot deal, new to the oncology world. His head was fitted with a metal contraption that looked like a small birdcage. He wore it for hours on the day of radiation treatment.

The radiation was a large dose but specifically aimed at the tumor site in the brain. It was meant to clean up any little (or big) residue from the surgery.

"Aren't you worried about losing brain cells?" I asked him.

"Stop worrying about the little things," he said.

That was Bobby, carefree and happy-go-lucky. It made me crazy.

Bobby said, "You should just worry about whether I'm going to live or die."

That did it. That put me over the edge.

I ran out of the hospital, getting lost in the parking garage. It took me an hour to find my car. I went straight home, locked the door, pulled down the shades, climbed into bed, and cried.

"What have I done?"

"What am I doing?"

Consider journaling about a time when you were so engrossed in an activity that you lost track of time. Does the memory of it bring back that good feeling? That good feeling is your own special flow.

Now write about the opposite: a time when you imposed control—either in your own life or the life of another. How did you feel then? How did it turn out for you?

PART FOUR

PIVOTING

Whatever makes you uncomfortable is your biggest opportunity for growth.
—Bryant McGill

People Pleaser

When you say "Yes" to others, make sure you are not saying "No" to yourself.
—Paolo Coehlo

Are you a people pleaser?

Perhaps you know one?

Or maybe you're married to one?

I'm a people pleaser and have been for decades. I fit the textbook definition.

The number one characteristic is seeking approval or validation from others. People pleasers almost never consider looking for validation from within. We want to be recognized and accepted by everyone. People pleasers need to feel needed.

When this behavior gets out of control, it's officially known as dependent personality disorder, more commonly known as codependency.

You can recognize a people pleaser by these traits:

- difficulty setting boundaries;
- denies or avoids conflict;
- low self-esteem;
- feels responsible for others;
- can't say no;
- remains in broken relationships;

- won't ask for help;
- cares too much what other people think.

This is not a comprehensive list. I've only included the traits that I know I've exhibited.

People pleasers offer apologies when none are necessary. You may agree (even if you do it yourself) that one of the most annoying traits is when the word "sorry" occurs every third or fourth sentence.

When I was in my 30s, my counselor said, "I'd like to see you start taking care of yourself before you take care of everyone else. We'll work on setting boundaries, saying no, and raising your self-esteem. This will help you overcome your codependency."

Whew. Really?

• • •

Tomas and I planned a month-long road trip to see family and friends, taking us through five states. We jokingly told each other we were doing this "while we can." You never know what the future holds. After that, we would continue on to Seaside, Oregon, for our usual summer break.

But with the diagnosis of stroke-related balance loss, I had some doubts about traveling in my wobbly condition. I went to see my doctor. She had been instrumental in getting to the bottom of my balance issues, ordering MRIs of my brain, getting me in to see a neurologist, and requesting physical therapy.

The medical assistant took my blood pressure. It was high.

Must be nerves, I thought.

Doctor Sarah walked in. I noticed she was wearing cute shoes with khaki pants and her crisp white doctor's coat. She got right to the point.

"How can I help you?"

"Tomas and I are planning a road trip through five states. I wanted to check in with you first."

My record of falls included two with head injuries—but fortunately no concussion. And even after many sessions of physical therapy, certain moves still made me feel off-balance and hesitant.

"I'm still wobbly. I'm still having trouble walking backwards, stepping in a circle backwards, and raising my arms while walking."

To prove it to herself, Dr. Sarah gave me her own routine of balance tests, two of which I failed. She looked at me.

"I can't release you for travel. Your fall risk is too great."

"What do you mean?" I panicked. "Is it because of my osteoporosis?"

"No," she said. "Your biggest risk is falling and sustaining a head injury."

She proceeded to describe all the head injuries I could incur, the worst being a brain bleed. She told me of another patient who'd sustained a brain bleed, resulting in blindness and dementia. His life changed forever. And it all started with a fall.

"You're a fall risk," she repeated. "I recommend you don't travel."

* * *

I left Dr. Sarah's office feeling anxious, sad, and nervous. I didn't want to tell my husband the doctor's verdict of "no travel." Not when Seaside had been our life every summer for the past seven years. And not when we had family expecting our visits.

I felt an ache in my collarbone. And I felt lightheaded.

After my nap, I still felt lightheaded—almost dizzy—and I started to sweat. The ache in my collarbone intensified.

I got in the car, and we went to pick up a prescription. By now I was sweating profusely and could feel nausea building. I rolled down the window for some fresh air. I was burning up. I peeled off my jacket and mopped my forehead.

We entered the drug store. I sat down on a bench at the entrance.

"You go ahead. I just need to sit here for a minute."

Holding the jacket I had shed, Tomas leaned down and looked me in the eye.

"Don't you think we should go to the ER?"

"Let me get some water," I stalled. "I'm probably dehydrated."

We left the store, walking arm in arm. His face showed worry mixed with terror.

"Are you sure about not going to the ER?"

"I'll be fine."

If I could just get home, drink some water, and lie down, I felt I could push through.

With rest and hydration, the symptoms did subside. But I had made a poor choice, and I knew better. When someone later asked me why I didn't go to the ER, I had a string of reasons.

"I didn't want to bother anyone, especially Tomas."

"It was nearly six o'clock, and we would miss dinner."

"I felt I could get this to pass without asking anyone for help."

"I feared a false alarm. I didn't want to inconvenience the doctors and nurses."

WTF??!!

That look of worry and terror on my husband's face haunted me. I never wanted to see that look again.

The Power of Getting Help

> Yesterday I was clever, so I wanted to change the world. Today I am wise, so I am changing myself.
> —Rumi

Today was the long-awaited day. I was finally going to decide where to hang some pictures in our townhouse.

After a big downsizing move, we finally felt settled enough to put up the artwork. Nearly a year had passed, and I was determined to get the art out of those boxes and onto the walls!

But something wasn't right.

I wasn't feeling well and had another bad headache. I'd had several in the previous few days. My blood pressure was also high. I normally never have headaches, and my blood pressure is almost always low.

I have a little spiral notebook. It's orange, and I got it for 98 cents. I like writing into my neat columns the date, the time, and the exact reading from the blood pressure machine that sits permanently on the coffee table. I record my blood pressure numbers morning and night.

You may recall from seeing a brochure or poster in your doctor's office that the ideal blood pressure for humans is 120/80. As long as you're somewhere near that mark, your blood pressure is considered normal.

Ever since my heart attack, I had prided myself on my low blood pressure.

"I'm medicated to read low," I'd say to the tech, who would comment on my low numbers.

I was on blood pressure medication and a beta blocker. Both are meant to help heart patients like me keep their numbers low. "It keeps the heart from working too hard," my pharmacist would say.

But now my reading was alarmingly high: 185/123.

My heart was pounding, and my head was throbbing. I was popping Aleve to quell the headache. I remembered what my friend, Jeannie, said about her racing heart: "It felt like there was a freight train in my chest." My heart was that freight train, and nausea rose in my throat.

What a nightmare. I tried to think. My brain wouldn't function.

Tomas was away for the day. I dialed his number. My call went to voicemail.

I started feeling anxious. High blood pressure is a precursor to stroke, and I knew that. I took my blood pressure again. Same. Way too high.

I texted Samantha, my cardiologist's nurse practitioner. She was the one person in the medical practice office I could always count on for help.

Sam: My BP is 185/123. Bad headache and nausea. Headache started three hours ago. I fear a stroke. I'm considering going to ER. Thoughts?

She texted back immediately.

I agree with you. Go. Keep me updated if you can.

I tried Tomas again. My call went straight to voicemail.

"Please, God," I prayed. "Have him here soon!"

Lying down on the soft red chenille sofa, I could barely lift my hurting head to put a small pillow under my neck. I closed my eyes. Even they hurt. I tried to distract myself by thinking pleasant thoughts. I thought about my mom and how she never seemed to get sick or show pain. My vision of her faded as a hammer kept pounding in my head.

Finally, I heard the garage door open. *Tomas is home!* I wanted to get up to greet him but feared any sudden movement would trigger fainting.

"Honey?" I barely squeaked it out. I'm pretty sure he didn't hear me.

"Honey, I need to talk to you."

Dropping his keys on the granite counter with a clang, he rushed to the sofa.

"What's wrong?"

"I'm having a problem."

Worry scrunched the skin on his forehead into wrinkles. "Tell me."

"I have the worst headache, my blood pressure is sky-high, and I'm afraid it might lead to a stroke."

"I'm calling Sam!" he said, reaching for his phone.

"I already texted her all the details. She says, go to the ER."

Tomas raised an eyebrow in surprise. "And you're okay with that?"

"Yes. Yes, I am. Let's go."

We filled a plastic grocery bag with a few things in case we had to stay over. As I maneuvered my body into the car, my head was pounding and my heart was racing.

"I'm calling Tim," Tomas said. All I could do was nod in agreement.

Tim's familiar voice came through on the car's Bluetooth speaker. "Hi, there. What's up?"

"We're on our way to TMC," Tomas told him.

"Oh, no. Mom? Are you okay? I can be there in fifteen minutes."

I wanted to tell him about my freight train, but I couldn't raise my voice enough to be heard. I whispered to Tomas, "Tell him I want him to come."

* * *

In the ER, the chilly waiting room was packed. Finally, an aide pushing a wheelchair came out to get me. She motioned for me to sit. Tim and Tomas followed us to Room 6, where she helped me onto the narrow bed.

A petite nurse in teal scrubs appeared. "I'm Brenda," she said, with a warm smile. Brenda had curly black hair and a cheerful manner. We learned that she's a travel nurse and she loves it.

She inserted an IV, then positioned the blood pressure cuff, the clip-on finger oxygen monitor, and electrodes for the EKG. As Brenda moved from one side of the bed to the other, she chatted with my husband and son, fielding their questions.

"I'm from Louisville. I started the travel nurse gig to help pay off my student loans. Yep, the pay is great."

A doctor came in to read my labs and EKG. "You can call me Dr. O," he said. "My name is hard to pronounce."

Dr. O looked at me. "When your sodium levels dip too low, it sends your body into a tailspin. I've ordered magnesium for your IV to bring up your sodium levels, and some pain reliever to help with the headache. You should feel better soon."

Hours passed. My thudding headache was gone, my blood pressure had dropped to 130/85, and I felt better. Now I was starving. Tim made a run to the cafeteria.

"Please bring me something salty!"

He returned with a bag of chips and a Sprite. "Oh, good! Give me those." I inhaled the chips.

Tomas stood and stretched, smiling sleepily. I knew he was relieved.

"Whatever was in that IV bag really worked," I marveled.

Brenda and Dr. O came in to say goodbye. "Anton will be here in a minute to go over your discharge papers," Dr. O informed me. "Remember to stay hydrated, okay?"

"I know, I know."

A different nurse came in. "You're about to be set free," Alison said with a laugh. "Brenda sent me in to unhook you."

She peeled the EKG stickers from my chest. Hearing someone behind her, she turned and said, "Oh, hi, Anton. She's ready for you."

Anton was tall and slim, with dark hair. He looked about 18. He had a computer on a rolling cart.

"Hello, I'm Anton. I'll get you checked out."

"Great," I said. "I'm starving. Let's go eat!"

Even though I knew I could walk, I found myself in another wheelchair. Alison pushed me to the lobby.

"Wait here," Tomas said. "I'll go get the car."

I noticed how empty the waiting room was. I looked out the plate-glass window and noticed how dark and empty the parking lot was. I had no idea what time it was. I had given Tomas my watch and phone.

Tomas pulled up to the curb. He gave me his hand and helped me out of the wheelchair and into the car.

"Finally! Let's get out of here! What time is it?" My heart sank as I looked at the digital clock on the dashboard: one-thirty a.m. "Oh, my gosh, no wonder I'm hungry! I don't care where we go. Let's just find a drive-thru."

We headed west on Grant, turning left on Craycroft. McDonald's was closed and dark.

"Let's try Wendy's," I said eagerly. "It's my favorite."

Driving two blocks, we could see the Wendy's was dark too.

"Aw, crap!"

"Don't worry, we'll find something," Tomas said. He pulled out his phone and did a quick search. "Aha! Burger King on Wilmot is open."

"Oh, thank goodness."

I had never been so hungry. I can't even tell you what I ate from Burger King because I downed it so fast.

We stumbled through the kitchen door at two-thirty. I was exhausted but happy because I felt so much better. The nightmare was over.

"Honey, will you help me get into bed? My legs aren't moving too well."

He put his arm around me. "Sure. Just lean on me."

Can you remember a time when you allowed yourself to get help and it ended up being a relief—instead of the thing you were dreading? Tell yourself this story in writing to find out what else it might reveal.

PART FIVE

WHAT'S A HEART REALLY FOR?

You are led through your lifetime by the inner learning creature, the playful spiritual being that is your real self.
—Richard Bach

Miles of Smiles

A smiling face is a beautiful face.
A smiling heart is a happy heart.
—Dr. T.P. Chia

I remember when I learned to smile. I was a lanky, gawky teenager with acne and cat's-eye glasses that were always crooked on my nose.

I loved *Seventeen*, a popular magazine for teen girls, and always read it from cover to cover. I adored the pretty models, the cute clothes, and the hairstyles diagrammed in the back section.

One day, I learned a life-altering secret on page 45.

I was about to enter junior high, which meant meeting lots of new kids from six or seven elementary schools. I desperately wanted to look like the girls in the magazine, but I had a few things holding me back.

First, I knew I had to get rid of my glasses and graduate to contact lenses. Next, my skin needed a miracle to become smooth and creamy, like the skin of the models in *Seventeen*. Last, I wanted to be popular. I wanted everyone to like me. Page 45 held the secret to my desires.

Number one on the list of "How to Be Popular" was simple but profound: *Smile at everyone. Smile all the time.*

So, I practiced.

And I had a great role model: Karen's big sister. She was a cheerleader in high school, and she had the biggest smile I'd ever seen. She smiled *all the time*. I even imagined her smiling in her sleep.

* * *

I convinced my mom to get me contact lenses, and to help me get rid of the horrible acne.

I was thrilled to learn she had booked me in with an optometrist and a dermatologist on the same day. I told all my friends. I was so sure that, by the next morning at John Marshall Junior High, I would be walking around my new school with pretty eyes and a clear face. *Voila!* I'd be transformed.

Little did I know that these contacts (called hard lenses) were of the earliest design in the industry and were famous for being uncomfortable.

I quickly learned how to put them in and take them out. You were not to wear them more than two to three hours a day until your eyes got used to them. On that first day wearing them to school, my eyes were bright red, bloodshot, and tearing up constantly.

Then there was my skin. Dermatologists at that time had a method using ultraviolet light and dry ice. On my first visit, the doctor had the nurse put me on a table in a private exam room. She fitted me with plastic goggles, which were meant to keep the damaging rays from my eyes.

Next came a giant sunlamp. When she clicked it on, a bright light flooded the room. As she angled the lamp directly over my face, I was glad for the protective goggles. The light felt warm on my skin, getting hotter by the minute. She was back in only three minutes, explaining that new patients are given treatment in short stints and then work up to longer times.

She proceeded to rub dry ice all over my hot face, jolting my senses from extreme heat to extreme cold. She assured me that this dramatic change in temperature was part of the acne treatment. Lucky for me, I didn't see my face until that evening. I was shocked to see that it was bright red.

You can imagine my disappointment the next morning as I arrived at school. My face was even redder than my eyes. There was no turning back.

My friends huddled around me, all talking at once.

"What happened, Susan?!"

My face burned as I blushed.

Could I get any redder?

* * *

While I kept having hot and cold skin treatments, I discovered Noxema and Clearasil to cover pimples and red blotches. My eyes adjusted to the contact lenses, and I could finally wear them all day. They were tinted blue and made my eyes look pretty.

Best of all, I knew how to smile like a cheerleader.

Suddenly, my life improved. I volunteered to work in the office during first period as a proctor—a sort of glorified runner. This gave me a chance to read all the notes that mothers had written to get their kids excused from school. I read them all before delivering them to each classroom. The other kids saw me sailing through our school halls, delivering important messages to teachers.

I ran for class secretary. Everyone voted for me and cheered me on. I won! I joined the drama club and tried out for parts in the plays. And I made the cut for choir. With my low voice, I was an alto.

One day I saw a notice in the school office from the local YMCA. They were hosting cheerleader classes. Real high school cheerleaders holding weekly clinics. Gasp!! I was determined to sign up and learn all the moves so I could be a cheerleader in high school. This became my burning ambition.

Guess what the head cheerleader, Sharon, said at the first class?

"Okay, girls, listen up! First and foremost, you have to learn to smile. I mean a really big smile that doesn't just fade away. Keep it on your face for the entire game!"

The other girls tried but couldn't hold the smile face nearly as long as I could.

I kept attending the clinics and classes until I had mastered all the jumps: the stag jump, the basic hurdle, the leaning backwards jump, and the splits jump. I learned to call out the cheers in my loudest, deep and booming voice, and then I mastered the giant pom-poms. Then there was the kneeling squat—hands on hips, and with a straight spine—to be used whenever silence was required at a game, such as during basketball free throws. I learned to jump-skip as I ran out on the field, and then cartwheel after skipping, all while smiling constantly.

I knew it all. I just had to make it through tryouts.

At North High School, cheerleading tryouts finally came true in my sophomore year. Twenty of us sat on the long bench at the center of the auditorium. Because my last name began with W, I was the last to be called. I was so nervous. It was agony watching 19 other girls perform cheers, jumps, and twirls.

When I heard my name called, I ran out onto the hardwood basketball floor, a gigantic smile plastered on my face. I called out "Ray Rah Red!" and the crowd chanted in time with my rhythmic arm movements. "Ray Rah White. Come on, Redskins, fight, fight, fight!" I leaped into the air, jumping my highest hurdle jump. I jumped a second one just as high. The crowd roared.

Afterwards, I had almost no recollection of my performance, only the chanting of the crowd.

The judges leaned over their clipboards. After long moments of waiting, the principal walked to the microphone to announce next year's cheerleaders. My heart was pounding.

Among the six chosen, there were only two sophomore names: mine and Paula's.

Later, I was told my smile made my performance special.

* * *

Winning an exciting contest was just the start of a lifetime of smiling.

I like to recall all the times a winning smile helped me out: job interviews, calling on clients, meeting new people, networking events. And, my favorite: interacting with children. From babies to toddlers to teens, a smile is guaranteed to cut through any shyness or wall they may have erected.

During my years as a single woman, I had plenty of dates, a few marriage proposals, and lots of fun. One evening out with girlfriends, they asked me the best way to meet a man.

"Smile at every man you meet. When you meet a guy you really like, turn your smile up to High. This means you're smiling with your lips but also adding a smile from your eyes, which is really from your heart."

Smiling even has proven health benefits. A study by psychological scientists found that participants who were asked to smile had lower heart rates after recovering from stressful activities.

But you won't need a scientific study to prove that smiling makes you feel better!

Be on the lookout for times when your own smile will make you feel better or enhance your life. Smile for no reason and see what comes of it.

Joie de Vivre

> Take those moments when something affects you deeply, or tickles your fancy, or piques your curiosity, to give in and allow your Inner Child to explore. NO judgments, no role-playing, no need to impress. No adulting by modern standards.
> —Runa Pigden

When I was little, I loved watching my mom pour milk into my small cup. When it was poured just right, it created a ring of magical bubbles.

"Oh, look!" she'd exclaim, pointing at the bubbles. "That means good luck and money in your future."

She'd clap her hands with glee, and I'd clap and giggle.

Little sister Sally would raise her cup with both hands. "Me, too, Mommy. Me, too!" And then, peering into her cup, she said, "I've got bubbles!"

"Do it again, Mommy!" we would cry out in unison.

Mom would pour steaming-hot coffee into her china cup.

"Oh, I'm lucky, too!"

She'd clap her hands and do a little jig around the table.

Hearing excited voices, Daddy would come find us. "What's all the giggling about?"

"Mommy poured money in my milk!"

A playful grin would brighten Daddy's face. "Pour me some, too!"

Mom would fetch another china coffee cup from the cabinet. Setting it gently before him, with her little girls watching intently, she'd lift the coffee pot and pour the steaming liquid.

"Now Daddy has bubbles, too!"

"Daddy, that means money! You have good luck!"

We'd laugh and clap our hands.

* * *

Mom loved all the children in her life. Grandchildren brought a new round of joy. Watching her entertain them was contagious fun. They had their favorite games.

"Grandma, do the red slipper dance!" they would beg. "Please! Please!"

Grandma Esther would disappear for a suspenseful minute. When she waltzed back into the room, my boys would squeal with delight.

"Watch the red slippers!" Timmy would cheer.

Timmy and Nathan were always mesmerized, and so was I. Grandma Esther would slowly move her feet as she started to hum.

"Old McDonald had a farm. . . ."

Her feet would shuffle forward and backwards, making a dance routine as she turned in a circle.

The kids would sing out "E-I-E-I-O!"

Grandma would laugh and clap her hands with joy.

Timmy and Nathan would clap, too. Pretty soon, everyone was singing the next part:

With a quack-quack here,
And a quack-quack there,
Here a quack, there a quack,
Everywhere a quack-quack!

Clapping, singing, dancing. Clapping, singing, dancing.

"Grandma, now dance to 'Wheels on the Bus'!"

Tim would glow with pleasure as he sang the familiar words:

The wheels on the bus go round and round, round and round.

Grandma Esther would then dance a different dance, a kind of two-step jig, still turning in a circle. Nathan would join her, hopping on his tiny feet and flapping his arms like a bird. He'd sing out *Round and round, round and round!*, and then fall down laughing on the floor.

Still dancing, Grandma would clap her hands in sheer delight.

Holding his arms out, Timmy would say, "Look at me!" Spinning in a circle, he'd laugh: "I'm diiiizzy!"

Falling into a breathless heap, Timmy would huff and puff the words "Round and round!" while watching for his favorite part—Grandma clapping with glee.

• • •

Mom took great joy in solving puzzles and writing jingles. During the 1950s, many contests invited consumers to try a product and then write something catchy, such as a rhyming jingle of 25 words or less.

One time, a famous company put on a contest for a new snack cracker. This was right up Mom's alley, and she couldn't wait to play the game. After reading the contest directions, she nibbled the end of her pencil, staring up at the ceiling.

"Hmm," she mused. "What would you name a tasty, bite-size cracker that could also be a name for a pony?"

After only a few moments of reflection, her face lit up.

"Why, Tidbit, of course!"

A few weeks later, an 18-wheeler came to a stop in front of our white stone ranch-style home at 1664 N. Clarence. Up and down the street, squealing kids poured out of their houses, swarming the huge truck that said Red Ball Freight on the side.

The driver, cap in hand, said, "Delivery for Esther Womer."

Daddy called out from the front door. "Esther?!"

"Mommy, Mommy!" we cried, crowding around her as the driver handed her a paper. "What is it? What is it?"

Staring down at the bill of lading, Mom's eyes were wide with wonder. Dropping the paper, she clapped for joy, shrieking, "Oh, girls, we have a piano!"

With a *ka-thump*, the driver and his helper put down a big steel ramp.

"Outta the way!" they yelled.

We stared in disbelief as an upright piano rolled down the ramp onto our driveway. It was made of beautiful blonde wood.

"Where to, ma'am?"

Mommy gathered my hand in her left and Sally's in her right.

"Follow us!" she said.

It fit perfectly against the wall next to the back picture window.

She didn't let go of our hands. We all just stood there and smiled.

* * *

The Turkey Creek Camp schedule came in the mail.

"Mom, Mom!" I said, pointing to the brochure. "Here's the session I want!"

It was my first sleep-away camp. I was 10.

One day after lunch we were on the singing porch, learning the words to "Make New Friends." I can still sing it.

Make new friends, but keep the old.
One is silver, and the other gold.

"Mail call!" said Pepper, a camp counselor. "Susan Womer?"

She placed a big, flat box in my outstretched hands.

"Boy, somebody got some goodies!" she grinned.

I cradled the box in my arms and walked back to my four-person tent in Sleepy Hollow.

Reading Mom's letter, my eyes filled with happy tears.

Dear Susan,

We miss you here at home, but we know you are having a wonderful time. Here's some writing paper and self-addressed, stamped envelopes. I can't wait to read your letters.

Love,
Mom

The box was filled with layers. My tentmates gathered around.

"Oh, boy, the Sunday comics!" Janie said, peering over my shoulder. "I love reading those!"

Under the folded comics was a flat layer packed neatly in wax paper. "My favorite cookies!" I shouted. "Snickerdoodles!"

But the bottom layer was the best.

"I'll sure never run out of candy or gum," I said to myself breathlessly. Specially-wrapped pieces of bubblegum were visible in the bottom layer. "Oh, my favorite!"

Only Mom could guess my favorite. It was Super Bubblegum, wrapped in a waxy, red-and-blue wrapper and twisted on the ends. I unwrapped one and popped it in my mouth. Between chews, I shared my opinion with Linda and Marilyn.

"So much better than Double Bubble or Bazooka!"

Next were Tootsie Rolls, those chocolatey, chewy candies. Also, Tootsie Roll Pops—all in cherry flavor—and rolls and rolls of Life Savers, also in cherry.

Mom had not forgotten my most favorite of all: Sugar Daddies! Milk caramel pops on a stick. I loved sucking on them with their sweet flavor. As I told Janie, "You can make one of these last all day."

"Oh, Mom," I sighed, as I imagined her putting the box of goodies together.

Our counselors rang the big bell at the lodge. We heard them calling out "Rest Period!" Some of the girls napped or rested. I spent the time writing a special letter.

Dear Mom,

Thank you so much for the gift box. I shared the comics with Janie, Linda, and Marilyn.

We share a tent. We are in Sleepy Hollow. That's the name of our spot in the camp. I love it here!

Love,
Susan

I visualized Mom joyfully opening and reading my letter. I pictured her reading it to Daddy and my sisters in her most gleeful voice. I could hear her clapping and see her thrilled smile. I knew she was already thinking of the next box of goodies she could pack for me.

Besides Mom, my Aunt Muriel was a perfect example of joie de vivre. She visited our home often. We felt an exciting swish of air whenever she entered the house. She would call out to the room, "Oh, my stars and garters! It's a beautiful day to be alive!" We would run to the door, hugging her and jumping around her with delight.

Recall a person (or a pet) in your own life who's filled with joy. What effect does this have on you and those around you? Put this in writing as a way to light up your world—and to bring a smile to the faces of those who know this pet or person, too.

My Inner Kid

> Play is the highest expression of human development in childhood, for it alone is the free expression of what is in a child's soul.
> —Friedrich Froebel

I'm a Kansas girl.

After moving to Arizona in my 20s, I found myself flying back and forth. When they both faced health challenges, my parents needed me.

I became quite familiar with the Wichita airport. I learned that the gift shop was a treasure trove of gifts, mementos, and toys. I always lingered at the toy display because the toys were so unique. Each one represented a famous character from Kansas history.

The best treasure I bought there was a set of dolls from *The Wizard of Oz*. They looked just like the characters from the original movie, filmed in 1939: Dorothy, Tin Man, the Cowardly Lion—and precious little Toto in Dorothy's basket.

These were not the kinds of dolls you'd find in the average toy store. They were not really play dolls but more like museum pieces or models for a diorama scene.

After I flew home to Tucson, I found the perfect woven basket with a curved handle, just like Dorothy's. Like miniature mannequins, I placed my new dolls in the basket. They looked so happy, just like a family gathered for a story. I placed this sweet arrangement on the hearth of my fireplace. I loved gazing at it, and I quickly learned that children were equally enchanted.

The dolls looked too fragile for games, but I didn't want to deprive any child of the pleasure of playing with them. Whenever I told kids they could take them out of the basket, they were always handled with great care.

Even decades later, I still smile as I visualize the threesome skipping along on a journey to the magic Emerald City, as the famous song "We're Off to See the Wizard" plays in my head.

* * *

On another trip to Kansas, I picked up a set of dolls based on the Lollipop Guild from *The Wizard of Oz*. They were so cute on their own, but when you placed them on the molded plastic form, they were planted in the Lollipop Forest.

Once, my girlfriend invited me over while her four-year-old granddaughter was visiting. I packed up the Lollipop Guild and arrived at her door. The little girl, Lacey, was infatuated.

"Do you like to make up stories about your toys?" I asked her.

"Yeeesssss!"

Lacey said she wanted to try it with the Lollipop Guild. We sat on the floor. I put two on my side and gave her two. I put the molded stand between us.

"Are you ready to go on an adventure?"

"Yippee!"

I pointed to the molded stand and named it Happy Home Island. That's the one place the dolls could go whenever they wanted to. To venture to other places, they had to ask permission.

I asked Lacey to show me the playground with the swings and slides. With her finger, she drew a circle on the rug.

"I think there may be a sidewalk leading to the toy store downtown," I said. "Do you know where it might be?"

She pointed to my left side. "Over there!"

We made up place after place for our make-believe town. We would take our Lollipop figurines to the playground, moving them forward in little hops, and then to the toy store, and then to the ice cream shoppe, and all the other wonder-filled places. Lacey's dolls' favorite was the slide on the playground. Each time we went to the playground, the slide became taller and taller, giving her dolls the thrill of their lives.

With a hop, skip, and a jump, the Lollipop Guild would always return to Happy Home Island.

* * *

I love kids.

I'm the one who will hold the crying baby while Mom goes to heat up a bottle. I'm the one who wanders away from the tour group to smile at the toddler who waved at me.

"Baby alert!" I often hear. "Tell Susan there's a baby in the room."

My husband even began approaching mothers with babies.

"My wife will give you a dollar if you let her hold your baby."

Ha! Funny, not funny.

At first I blushed with embarrassment, but then I realized he was right. Every time he does it, I'm in heaven. My heart leaps as I catch Baby's eye, and he gives me a big smile. When I'm near enough to smell him, I inhale the sweet scent of soap, baby powder, and soft flannel blankets.

When I finally get the hand-off from her arms to mine, he fits snugly into the crook of my arm. I can bring the top of his head to my cheek and brush that soft fluff of fuzz back and forth.

Next, I bring in the finger games, such as "Itsy-Bitsy Spider" and tickle monster. If Baby's feet are exposed, I bring in some toe games, feeding my affection for sweet baby toes. I love to look at any baby's feet, seeing tiny loaves of bread, or puffy biscuits with toes added for fun.

Toddlers' toes are priceless, too. Whenever I see a photo of a barefoot toddler, or watch one at play, I adore seeing that upward lift of the big toe when they're deep in concentration.

For me, holding a baby or playing with a toddler is even more relaxing than a spa-day pedicure or foot massage.

• • •

Charlie was a gift from a friend. He was adorable, and he made me smile.

Charlie was a stuffed bear with spots more like a leopard than a bear. He sported a gold bow at his neck. Little did I know Charlie would become Patrick's favorite stuffed animal.

Patrick is my first-born grandson. When I describe the joy of being a grandparent, I like to say, "A tiny human steals your heart when you least expect it!"

I volunteered to babysit. Having Patrick in my home every Saturday made my week complete.

For playtime, I collected some children's books from my favorite bookstore and mixed my collection of display dolls with his Tonka trucks, his stuffed bunny, and his miniature wooden train set.

We made up stories with fun settings, from an elevator in a 10-story building to an amusement park where we could slide on the backs of dinosaurs. We could even catapult ourselves to fly through the clouds.

After gathering Charlie, my Tin Man, the Lollipop Guild, and his Thomas the Tank Engine, Patrick would ask me to join them on a trip to the "magic office" on the top floor of the Bentley Building. With all the appropriate *whooshing* noises, we would ride the elevator to the top floor, holding our tummies all the way. The elevator ride always made our tummies jump up to our throats.

The best part was naptime. This was when he could pick out two books. I would read one, and he would read the second one. I would pretend to fall asleep as he was reading. Patrick would snuggle Charlie Bear to my cheek and lay his head down next to mine. And then he would drift off. It's one of my sweetest memories.

As I write this book, Patrick is 21. But, back then as a little guy, he reminded me that taking the time to play and practice make-believe can whisk away my troubles and put my rushing brain on pause.

Have you seen the vast range of coloring books for grownups? Some say coloring induces the same inner state as meditating, by quieting the activity of a restless mind.

Rewarding My Heart

Just do the simple acts of love for yourself, and then your authentic self begins.
—Anonymous

I grew up with rewards for accomplishments.

Our family celebrated A's on report cards, sports and contest wins, graduations, and more. Mom even threw a party when her grandson got his driver's license. I couldn't help but follow in her footsteps.

Eventually, celebrating others gave way to rewarding myself for adult accomplishments. Rewards of favorite foods changed to favorite drinks.

By my late 20s, I loved the sweet and salty taste of margaritas, either over ice or blended to a cool, sweet slush and served in a giant goblet. One tequila-drenched drink was enough to put a smile on my face, washing away the stress and tension of a long, hard workweek.

As I moved up the corporate ladder, my officemates became the executives of the company—mostly men. After-work drinks were either poured in the executive suite or at the oak-paneled bar in the lobby of our 12-story office building. This was the 1980s.

I ordered what the men were drinking: gin and tonic, whiskey on the rocks, martinis, and manhattans. The drinks still made me smile and eased the tight muscles in my shoulders. But soon I had to admit that these end-of-week gatherings were causing me stress of another kind.

As one of the few women invited into this group, I had to conserve my energy, which was the tool I used to level the playing field with the men during the workday. It was exhausting. I started cutting back on my happy hours and heading home. Once there, I could be my own bartender and pour a drink of my choosing. I bounced from cabernet and chardonnay to beer, from vodka to bloody marys, and then back to my old standby, the margarita.

Even though I usually felt relaxed after the first one, to justify a second drink—another "reward"—I often told myself, "You deserve it." By then I was in my 40s, single, and enjoying my freedom. I was working so hard for my success, and to make a name for myself, that my schedule left little time for positive self-care practices.

Or so it seemed.

Interestingly, I still found time for more rewards.

I discovered the home shopping network. I especially liked watching the jewelry segments. Soon, I had my own account and secret number to get through to the host. I heard myself on TV, chatting about the products. I became hooked on this new form of relaxation.

Eventually, I gave up TV shopping for bricks-and-mortar department stores. My favorites were on the high end: Nordstrom, Saks, and Neiman Marcus. Tucson was a smaller city, so I had to drive to Phoenix to shop in those stores.

Dillard's was right in my neighborhood, and the designer clothes were on the second floor. I learned I could drive to the mall, pull in the side entrance, find the ramp to the upper level, and park right at the door. By going in the upper entrance, I could get right to shopping for all my favorite brands.

I would cruise the racks, plucking out items I liked and draping them over my forearm. By the time my arm was aching, I would either find a dressing room or simply check out. I knew I could always try everything on at home.

My closets bulged with pretty clothes, but the excitement I felt in the store always faded by the next day. Even so, I kept going back to shop. After all, it was my reward for hard work.

My credit card balances were rising every month. I began to recognize that addictively treating myself was counterproductive to my efforts to build a retirement account.

I needed a better reward.

* * *

I started attending a yoga class and loved it.

I attended three times a week and felt the benefits of the restorative poses, such as child's pose, pigeon pose, and corpse pose. I lost a few pounds, even as I gained muscle strength in my legs and core.

I also began doing stretches at home, enjoying the rewards of moving my body.

One day, a substitute instructor led our yoga class. She did the poses in a different order, and then led us in a five-minute meditation. In just five minutes, I floated away. That feeling was the best reward I'd given myself in years. Better than any margarita.

I kept meditating and loved the stillness of it. The stillness felt like praying, and a little bit like daydreaming. When I drew from that well of peace and quiet, I felt calm.

I decided stillness was good for me, good for my head, and especially good for my heart.

* * *

By that time in my life, my job and the corporate environment were the most demanding I had ever experienced. I believed that the stress and the draining schedule would be worth it in the long run, as long as I could withstand it physically and emotionally. I knew the income from the next few years would provide a financial future for myself and my family, so I made that my challenge.

I noticed how depleted my energy would get from social interactions, business meetings, and loan committee. I used to come home from work, plop down on my sofa, and say, "I can't talk to one more person!"

I set out to create some alone time for myself. Fortunately, I had a flexible schedule at work. I could come and go from the office and still generate new business for loans and take care of my existing customers.

I took off early on Tuesdays and Thursdays for my yoga class. I could take the time to spend a day at home, doing anything or nothing. I found solace in wandering museum exhibits and antique stores. I was a regular at my favorite bookstore.

Old classic movies played every afternoon at two-thirty. Sometimes I left the office for a movie and an afternoon nap on my comfy sofa. For deeper rejuvenation, I could check into a health spa for a day or a weekend.

Some weekends, when the sky was overcast and I wanted to stay in, I loved going through Mom's old photo albums. Her distinctive handwriting named every person in each photo. I also had Grandma Gracie's diaries. These were bound in leather, with a latch that locked. One could write about two inches in the small space for each day. It was a five-year diary, so I could indulge in years of history.

Visiting a florist shop would trigger my senses with the glorious colors and heady aromas. I also loved touring the local nursery. I would plant flowers twice a year. First, I'd spend an entire day organizing my workspace. It was like an assembly line: potting soil, plant fertilizer, rows of pots, and flats of colorful flowers.

The best part was filling the pot with soil, carefully lifting the small square of roots, stems, and petals from the flat, and then placing it in a perfectly-sized hole. My fingers would gently tamp down the soil around the delicate seedlings. Working with the beauty of flowers and the earthiness of potting soil reconnected me to myself.

I learned the hard way (and more than once) that my heart needs relief and revitalization. Instead of fleeting rewards, I can fill my heart with joy and color, or with peace and stillness.

What are some authentic rewards you love that would nurture your heart? Explore these in writing to remind yourself what you've been missing. You may be surprised by how many heart-nourishing things you write down once you get in the flow. Don't forget to include fun things. Fun is good medicine. When your list is done, don't wait! Choose the simplest one first and give yourself that treat.

PART SIX

THE TRUE SELF

Your heart speaks to you through your feelings deep within. If you follow your heart, your life will undoubtedly change. You will be guided by your true self, instead of what you think you should do.
—Niki Banas

Heart in Nature

> The goal of life is to make your heartbeat match the beat of the universe, to match your nature with Nature.
> —Joseph Campbell

In Bible study, my young friend asked me an insightful question.

"How do you know when God is near you?"

After a moment of contemplation, I said, "I feel him in the breeze. I hear him in the rushing waters. I sense his presence when I inhale the scent of evergreen trees."

Nature fills my heart with wonder and awe.

Growing up in Kansas, I witnessed Mother Nature flaunting her classic beauty in every car trip across the state. In summer, we'd pass fields of wheat awaiting harvest. I was mesmerized as the breeze rippled the yellow-gold stalks. I was positive the line from "America the Beautiful" about *amber waves of grain* referred to our Kansas wheatfields.

To clear up a myth, Kansas isn't always flat. Striking rock formations stand up proudly, such as Castle Rock and Monument Rocks. The Flint Hills are gently rolling hills of tallgrass prairie. Kansas even has its own mountains, the highest of which is Mount Sunflower.

In my hometown of Wichita, two rivers converge. That confluence is marked by a beautiful park with trails, special lighting, and speakers playing a recorded history of the area. Standing proudly on a boulder is a majestic bronze statue of a Native American—arms raised, head tilted to the sky, headdress fanning, and the fringes of his pants ruffled by the breeze—known as *The Keeper of the Plains*. As the Little Arkansas River joins the Big Arkansas River, this stately piece of art silently watches over the crashing waters.

Decades later, I watched the mighty Columbia River flow into the Pacific Ocean at the South Jetty in Warrenton, Oregon. Looking out over the huge jetty rocks, I saw a line of seething water where the river and the ocean meet. I couldn't take my eyes off of it. The force of the currents clashing was so powerful, I felt it in my spirit.

• • •

As teenagers, my friends and I attended weekly meetings of Young Life, a Christian-based organization reaching out to young people. Held in private homes, the meetings were fun, filled with singing songs and playing games.

I volunteered our house for meetings. Kids came from all over town, sitting cross-legged on our living room floor and listening to Pastor John uplift us. They passed pocket-sized songbooks with lyrics to popular Christian songs, and Chris played his guitar.

But the best part was the Young Life camp in Colorado. Spread across 20 acres, the camp featured a huge lodge, dining hall, log cabins, and horse stables. We were surrounded by pine forests and beautiful mountains.

Winter or summer, I went to as many camps as I could. I went so often that, the summer of my junior year, I qualified for a spot on the work crew. During my month on the work crew, we were assigned to work the jobs of waiter, cook, laundry detail, or cleaners of the guest cabins. There were around 25 of us, and we made friends from all over the country.

Each week, a new group of campers arrived on a bus filled with noisy teenagers. The new campers stayed for five days, giving us workers a two-day break in between sessions. As a treat during our breaks, the counselors took over our work duties.

Those lazy weekends were filled with horseback riding, swimming, and hiking. On one of our Saturdays off, we hiked up a curving trail to meet our counselors, Jim and Chris, at a clearing about a mile up. As we climbed the trail, the smell of pine was intoxicating.

In the clearing, we discovered a huge fire pit, with a grill the size of a fence gate. And there was Jim, cooking thick T-bone steaks, potatoes, and corn on the cob. The air was crisp, the campfire glowed, and Chris played his guitar. We raised our voices in song. By then, we knew all the words to every song in the songbook.

After darkness fell, more stars were visible in the sky than I'd ever seen, and the evening breeze began to stir. They were singing one of my favorite songs. I joined in.

Oh Lord, my God,
When I, in awesome wonder
Consider all the worlds Thy hands have made,

I see the stars, I hear the rolling thunder;
Thy power throughout the universe displayed.
Then sings my soul, my Savior God to Thee,
How great Thou art, how great Thou art.
Then sings my soul, my Savior God to Thee,
How great Thou art, how great Thou art.

As we sang the fourth and fifth lines—*I see the stars, I hear the rolling thunder; Thy power throughout the universe displayed*—my voice caught in my throat. It was then that I felt it. The evening breeze had turned to a light wind, brushing my cheek and lifting the hair off my neck.

I heard Counselor Jim talking softly, inviting us to let Jesus into our hearts. I looked up at the awe-inspiring night sky. My heart was as wide-open as the expansive sky of stars. When I felt the gentle wind touch my face, I knew it was the hand of God.

I felt his Spirit in the air, the sky, the trees, and the stars. It was easy to imagine him moving right into my heart, as softly as the breeze.

In your busy life, how can you get more time in nature? Maybe by including others?

Did you know that even seeing pictures of nature, or a tree through a window, can give you some of the same benefits? Try looking on YouTube—there's an abundance of videos showing heart-meltingly beautiful scenes from nature. Perhaps you could also rearrange some furniture, to give you a better view of your favorite tree from your favorite comfy chair.

If My Heart Ruled the World

> The human mind and what we've achieved with it is remarkable. But it does not come close to what we can do, be, see with our hearts.
> —Rasheed Ogunlaru

"I do everything the man does, only backwards and in high heels!"

I first heard this quote from legendary dance star Ginger Rogers at a women's conference. This was an all-day event filled with women speakers. There were also classes, each one designed to help us improve our position in the workplace or in the world.

The keynote speech was about being a woman in a man's world. I'll never forget the way the speaker strode to the podium, tapped the microphone, and then proceeded to rip up the duct tape holding the microphone cord to the floor.

"Now I can move around the stage with ease," she said, "speaking to everyone in the audience without the podium blocking your view of me. I am the dominant figure up here, not the podium!"

Her message was about just that—being the dominant one in the room, in the class, or in the company. She talked of standing up, standing out, and making an impression.

During that decade, the 1980s, I participated in seminars about setting goals and accomplishing them in a man's world. There was a movement afoot to get women up the corporate ladder to leadership positions, complete with equality in pay. I was fired up about this and ready to do my part, even pursuing senior-level corporate positions. I vowed to hire more women in roles where there was a path for growth.

This women's movement swept the nation, encouraging us working women to take on as much as we possibly could, while raising children, running a family, being an adoring wife and, of course, getting dinner on the table.

Near the end of this incredible period in my life, I had to seek counseling for a growing mental health issue among American women, known as Superwoman Syndrome. The condition can be defined like this:

Superwoman Syndrome occurs when a woman chronically neglects her own needs in her quest for perfection in all areas of her life—career, family, home, exercise, and social activities.

An insidious and deceptive idea prevailed: that fulfilling all of these roles to perfection would lead to feeling complete as a woman. Instead of feeling fulfilled, I found myself feeling stressed, anxious, and perpetually fatigued.

As we know today, the stress caused by trying to "do it all" can cause myriad health issues, such as early aging, diabetes, obesity, gastrointestinal conditions—and heart disease.

• • •

In *The Heart of Consciousness*, a book that highlights scientific advancements in neurocardiology, Mindie Kniss wrote: "The research is conclusive that the heart is a conscious organ."

What if we could direct the energy in our hearts to achieve a peaceful, loving world, where all beings are considered equal and children are treasured?

If my heart had its way, the world would change in a new kind of "Big Bang," with this loving force raising the consciousness of all beings it touched. Then, when we loved, when our own hearts reached out in tenderness, it would be a repeat of the greater cosmos reaching out with its heart.

If my heart ruled the world, power and conflict would be replaced by love and caring. All thoughts of war and disruption would vanish, and people would be pleasant and kind. We'd see a Statue of Liberty standing tall in every country and state, symbolizing welcome and freedom for every person entering.

My heart would start with the children. By providing education, nourishment, community, family support, and more exposure to nature, each child would feel loved and cherished. Each child would learn how to love others, in a world of peace, beauty in nature, and satisfying abundance.

This heartfelt society would ensure that each child started with a happy early learning experience, learning about living and playing with others. As each child progressed through the grades, he or she would be encouraged to embrace creativity, diversity, and family life.

As they advanced through each year of life, these children would deepen their understanding of love and world peace. These experiences would provide a natural curiosity about the world around them. This curiosity would spark joy in the hearts of family members, teachers, and mentors, and they would willingly provide answers to each child's questions and curiosities.

If my heart ruled the world, each child would experience gentle honesty and loving support from the adults in their lives. Adults would encourage opportunities to learn and create. That power of encouragement would stimulate imagination, the authentic self, and a deep connection to the heart.

As children matured into young adults, they would be granted the freedom to experience the climate and culture they most desired. This choice would place them in a world they were best suited to. There, they would develop the skills related to their deepest interests. Later, as content and well-adjusted adults, they would nurture and educate the next generation of children.

The cycles would grow and evolve, as each generation connected to the next from the heart.

Ponder what your own vision would be if your heart ruled the world. To get your imagination's engine running, close your eyes and daydream. Make it a big dream. Write it in your journal. When your future self reads it, you'll be amazed by what you envisioned.

The Heart's Wisdom

> Follow your heart and listen when it speaks to you.
> —Susanna Tamaro

After four years of surviving a heart attack, I desperately wanted to find my "new normal." Why was it so elusive? I think it was me trying to shape my life into a new normal that resembled my old normal.

One day, I decided to bring in my heart as a partner.

I remembered a technique a therapist had taught me. It involved talking to those parts of yourself that may be protecting you from uncomfortable feelings or long-ago trauma.

"It's all a matter of going within," he explained. "Call on the specific protector and have a talk."

That had worked well with my inner protectors, so I decided to try it with my heart.

At first, talking to my heart felt awkward, and I couldn't be sure she was listening. I realized I needed to relax. After relaxing, I felt less self-conscious. I started sharing things with my heart like I would with a friend, even talking out loud to her.

As I got used to it, I began to notice that she does reply—*if* I give her the space to do that. Her replies are usually feelings or subtle whispers of intuition.

Eventually, I got around to the dreaded subject: looking for my new normal. I wanted my heart to guide me, so I wouldn't fall back into my old patterns. I was nervous. *How the heck do I do this?* Then one of those intuitive moments came, showing me that I needed to write about it.

I took a deep breath, and said, "Okay, Heart! Let's go!"

When I journaled using the words "my heart" and "my new normal," even more intuition kicked in. My mind flashed over many things that have brought me joy over the years, and I jotted them down as fast as I could. The list included babies, toddlers, kids, massages, pedicures, and old movies. With barely time for a breath, the list went on: flowers, sewing, making jewelry, and writing fiction.

I imagined my heart saying, "That's enough for now. Start with these, and then see how you feel."

Within three days, my spirits were lifted. I indulged in a massage, watched two old movies on TV, and enjoyed visiting my neighbor, who cares for her eight-year-old grandson.

That kid! He was used to getting attention by acting out. I bent down and spoke quietly.

"Why don't you tell me a secret story about the little people who live in the community pool area?"

His eyes grew wide. I started the story, and he finished it beautifully.

"Can we do this again?" he said, wriggling with eagerness.

"Sure thing!"

* * *

With one of her whispers of intuition, my heart pointed me back to my list. When I reviewed the list, I was reminded of one of my novels and its main character, Sally Claymore. Fiction writing is so fun!

Sally was a banker in the 1990s and the only female in her corporate world. It was a mystery, filled with robbery, fraud, intrigue, and love affairs. It had been 20 years since I'd worked on it.

That afternoon, I pulled out my novel and started writing a new chapter. The goal was to plunge Sally into a big dilemma. To my surprise, I was able to pick up right where I left off. What a thrill it was. I didn't realize the simple act of inventing a problem for a fictional character could bring me such joy.

This joyful state came with an added bonus. I got my confidence back! I had a spring in my step and a smile in my voice. I felt like I could take on the world.

"Maybe this is what 'normal' can feel like," I said to myself.

I couldn't wait to tell my heart.

"You were so right about doing even more of the things I love to do! Sally Claymore danced off the page and rekindled my imagination."

I pictured myself confiding this to her over a cup of tea. *Next time I'll bring scones*, I thought. Based on the warm glow in my chest, I believed I could feel my heart smiling.

"You know what else?" I said. "I'm going to use my sewing machine. It's been years!"

Later, feeling the machine's cool steel beneath my fingers and watching the needle move up and down put me into a trance.

"I'll cut this infinity scarf in half and make two scarves from the delicate silk," I told my heart as I worked. The fabric flowed between my hands, charming my sense of touch.

The next day, I was on fire to share my outcomes with her: "The scarves turned out beautifully. I gave one to my friend Kathleen and kept the other."

At the store, I bought three bunches of fresh-cut flowers—two for my house, and one for Melissa—as well as 4" pots of luscious geraniums. I was in heaven, repotting them into 8" clay pots for our cozy front porch.

The best part was opening the bag of potting soil. It had been sitting in the sun, so the dirt felt warm in my hands. I loved that old, familiar feeling of scooping it into the pots and patting around the roots.

I stood back to enjoy my handiwork.

"They're bright red, and they look so pretty!"

I knew my heart would agree. Bright colors and happy things to look at are food for the heart.

I felt inspired to try even more of my favorite things. I raided my mother's jewelry box and repurposed some of her vintage jewelry—so much more satisfying than buying something new! Moving through the house in a happy dream, I spotted my redbird collection. They're made of ceramic, glass, and porcelain. It was fun dusting and rearranging them, and then admiring them anew.

As I dusted, I remembered the list I'd made after my intuition nudged me. That's when something that seemed so obvious in hindsight hit me: *My heart isn't just* about compassion, self-love, or loving others—it's about passion for the things I love to do.

I wanted my heart to know the healing impact this was having on me.

"I feel really good now. The worries I had melted away. It was like the scales fell from my eyes."

Have you ever thought of talking with your heart? I invite you to plunge in. It will probably feel awkward at first, but I hope you'll give it a try. Remember to pause and listen, and then write down what your heart says to you. It will usually be a feeling or a subtle intuition.

ABOUT THE AUTHOR

Writing is my passion. I've been writing all my life. I wrote a book in fifth grade, and a neighborhood newspaper at age 10. I studied journalism in school, working as a team with my classmates to publish the student newspaper and yearbook. Over the years, I have contributed to many magazines, with interviews as my specialty. This was my side gig while working in the corporate world as a banker. I've shared my talents by teaching writing, hosting online workshops and writers' groups, and creating a handbook for beginning a memoir.

I'm a heart attack survivor, and a Mayo Clinic-trained women's heart health advocate. My mission is to spread the heart health message to other women, with a warning: "Don't do what I did. Know the symptoms. Know your body. And, slow down. Remember, you can't do anything if you're dead."

I feel this book is the most important thing I've ever written. I'm also a speaker, ardently addressing groups and gatherings about heart health. While pacing myself and staying hydrated, I'm also a blogger at susansmithheart.com.

I'm married to my best friend, Tomas, and we live in Tucson, Arizona. We spend summers in Seaside, Oregon. I love being with my family and friends.

Reading a good book, watching an old classic movie, and writing for fun are at the top of my hobby list. I also enjoy a deep dive into history. I appreciate Mother Nature and the beauty she gives us.

To contact the author:
susan@susansmithheart.com

You can find Susan online at:
susansmithheart.com

INTERVIEWS & HEART HEALTH RESOURCES

It's never too late to take your heart health seriously and make it a priority.
—Jennie Garth

The more women survivors I meet, the more I realize there are many different diagnoses for heart disease in women. Each woman has her own unique story.

I want to spread the word, so I've created a collection of video interviews entitled *Heart of the Matter*. The stories from 20 survivors cover a range, including congenital heart disease, open heart surgery, atrial fibrillation, heart transplant, and heart failure.

You can find these videos on my website under the Interviews tab.

When I talk with heart patients, I like to recommend books, blogs, online support groups, and medical resources. I post these on my website under the Resources tab.

Click on the Interviews or Resources tab at
susansmithheart.com

Made in United States
Troutdale, OR
10/07/2023